Tucholsky Wagner Zola Scott Sydow Freud Schlegel
Turgenev Wallace Fonatne
Twain Walther von der Vogelweide Fouqué Friedrich II. von Preußen
Weber Freiligrath Frey
Fechner Fichte Weiße Rose von Fallersleben Kant Ernst Frommel
Richthofen
Engels Fielding Hölderlin
Fehrs Faber Flaubert Eichendorff Tacitus Dumas
Eliasberg Ebner Eschenbach
Feuerbach Maximilian I. von Habsburg Fock Zweig
Ewald Eliot Vergil
Goethe London
Mendelssohn Balzac Shakespeare Elisabeth von Österreich
Lichtenberg Rathenau Dostojewski Ganghofer
Trackl Stevenson Doyle Gjellerup
Mommsen Tolstoi Hambruch
Thoma Lenz Hanrieder Droste-Hülshoff
Dach Verne von Arnim Hägele Hauff Humboldt
Karrillon Reuter Rousseau Hagen Hauptmann Gautier
Garschin
Damaschke Defoe Hebbel Baudelaire
Descartes Hegel Kussmaul Herder
Wolfram von Eschenbach Schopenhauer Rilke George
Bronner Darwin Dickens Grimm Jerome
Campe Melville Bebel Proust
Horváth Aristoteles
Bismarck Vigny Barlach Voltaire Federer Herodot
Gengenbach Heine
Storm Casanova Tersteegen Grillparzer Georgy
Chamberlain Gilm
Brentano Lessing Langbein Gryphius
Strachwitz Claudius Schiller Lafontaine
Kralik Iffland Sokrates
Katharina II. von Rußland Bellamy Schilling
Gerstäcker Raabe Gibbon Tschechow
Löns Hesse Hoffmann Gogol Wilde Gleim Vulpius
Luther Heym Hofmannsthal Klee Hölty Morgenstern
Roth Heyse Klopstock Puschkin Homer Kleist Goedicke
Luxemburg La Roche Horaz Mörike Musil
Machiavelli Kierkegaard Kraft Kraus
Navarra Aurel Musset
Lamprecht Kind Kirchhoff Hugo Moltke
Nestroy Marie de France
Nietzsche Nansen Laotse Ipsen Liebknecht
Marx Lassalle Gorki Klett Leibniz Ringelnatz
von Ossietzky May vom Stein Lawrence Irving
Petalozzi Knigge
Platon Pückler Michelangelo Kafka
Sachs Poe Liebermann Kock
de Sade Praetorius Mistral Zetkin Korolenko

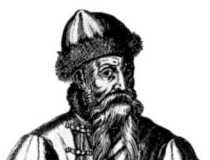

The publishing house tredition has created the series **TREDITION CLASSICS**. It contains classical literature works from over two thousand years. Most of these titles have been out of print and off the bookstore shelves for decades.

The book series is intended to preserve the cultural legacy and to promote the timeless works of classical literature. As a reader of a **TREDITION CLASSICS** book, the reader supports the mission to save many of the amazing works of world literature from oblivion.

The symbol of **TREDITION CLASSICS** is Johannes Gutenberg (1400 – 1468), the inventor of movable type printing.

With the series, tredition intends to make thousands of international literature classics available in printed format again – worldwide.

All books are available at book retailers worldwide in paperback and in hardcover. For more information please visit: www.tredition.com

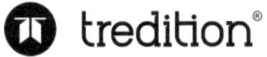

tredition was established in 2006 by Sandra Latusseck and Soenke Schulz. Based in Hamburg, Germany, tredition offers publishing solutions to authors and publishing houses, combined with worldwide distribution of printed and digital book content. tredition is uniquely positioned to enable authors and publishing houses to create books on their own terms and without conventional manufacturing risks.

For more information please visit: www.tredition.com

An Epitome of the Homeopathic Healing Art Containing the New Discoveries and Improvements to the Present Time

B. L. (Benjamin L.) Hill

Imprint

This book is part of the TREDITION CLASSICS series.

Author: B. L. (Benjamin L.) Hill
Cover design: toepferschumann, Berlin (Germany)

Publisher: tredition GmbH, Hamburg (Germany)
ISBN: 978-3-8495-1055-8

www.tredition.com
www.tredition.de

Copyright:
The content of this book is sourced from the public domain.

The intention of the TREDITION CLASSICS series is to make world literature in the public domain available in printed format. Literary enthusiasts and organizations worldwide have scanned and digitally edited the original texts. tredition has subsequently formatted and redesigned the content into a modern reading layout. Therefore, we cannot guarantee the exact reproduction of the original format of a particular historic edition. Please also note that no modifications have been made to the spelling, therefore it may differ from the orthography used today.

CONTENTS

AN EPITOME OF THE HOMŒPATHIC HEALING ART.

INTRODUCTION.

ADMINISTRATION OF REMEDIES.

DISEASES OF FEMALES

INDEX.

APPENDIX

TABLE OF REMEDIES.

In this table I have affixed to the remedies figures designating the dilutions or the attenuations, at which, under ordinary circumstances, I would advise their use. The strongest, or mother tinctures, marked with an apha (0), the dilutions or triturations to be of the decimal degrees of attenuation, are marked 1, 2, 3, &c., to designate that they are to be used at 1-10th, 1-100th, 1-1000th, &c., the strength of the pure drugs.

The list for a full Family Case contains all the remedies recommended in this book for diseases that may be safely trusted to unprofessional hands.

The Traveler's Case needs only such medicines as are prescribed for the diseases which he would be most liable to contract on his journey; though I have put in the principal ones used in domestic practice, so that the Case will do for family use.

The Cholera Case is only supplied with such remedies as are particularly applicable to that disease; useful, however, for many other complaints.

TRAVELER'S CASE.

1 Aconite	p 3	15 Hydrastus Can.	p 1
2 Apis Mellifica	p 3	16 Ipecac	p 3
3 Arsenicum	p 3	17 Mercurius sol.	p 3
4 Arnica	tr 0	18 Mercurius cor.	tt 2
5 Arum triphyllum	tt 2	19 Macrotin	tt 1
6 Belladonna	p 3	20 Nux Vom.	p 3
7 Baptisia	p 1	21 Phosphorus	p 3
8 Bryonia	p 3	22 Phos. acid	p 3
9 Colocynth	p 3	23 Podophyllin	p 2
10 China Sul.	tt 1	24 Rhus toxicod.	p 3
11 Chamomilla	p 3	25 Secale	p 3
12 Copaiva	p 2	26 Tartar emetic	p 3
13 Cuprum	p 3	27 Veratrum	p 3
14 Eupatorium Aro.	p 1		

CHOLERA CASE.

1 Aconite	p 3	8 Laurocerasus	p 4
2 Arsenicum	p 3	9 Opium	p 3
3 Belladonna	p 3	10 Merc. cor.	p 3
4 Camphor	tr 0	11 Phosphorus	p 3
5 Carbo Veg.	p 5	12 Phos. acid	p 3
6 Cuprum	p 3	13 Secale	p 3
7 Ipecac	p 3	14 Veratrum	p 3

[Pg 4]

FULL FAMILY CASE.

Tr. is used for tincture, Tt. trituration, P. pellets.

REMEDIES.	CONTRACTIONS.	
1 Aconitum.	Aconite	Tr 0 1 p 3
2 Althæa.		
3 Apis mellifica.	Apis mel.	0 p 2 3
4 Arsenicum.	Arsenicum	0 p 3
5 Arnica.	Arnica,	0 p 3
6 Arum triphyllum.	Arum triphyllum,	0 tt 2
7 Belladonna.	Bell.	tr 1 p 4
8 Baptisia tinctoria.	Baptisia,	tr 0 2
9 Bryonia.	Bryonia,	tr p 3
10 Carbo. Vegetabilis.	Carbo. Veg.	tr p 4
11 Cantharides.	Cantharides,	tr 0 p 3
12 Colocynthis.	Colocynth,	tr or p 3
13 China Sulphuricum.	China Sul.	tt 1
14 Chamomilla.	Chamomilla	tr or p 3
15 Copaiva.	Copaiva	tr 1 p 2
16 Cauloph. Thalictroides.	Caulophyllum	tr 1
17 Cuprum.	Cuprum,	p 3
18 Cuprum Aceticum.		
19 Cornus Sericea.	Cornus sericea, tr 0 p 2	
20 Conium maculatum.	Conium mac.	0 p 3
21 Coffea.	Coffea	p 4
22 Eryngium Aquaticum.	Eryngium Aquaticum	2
23 Eupatorium aromaticum	Eupatorium aro. tr 0 p 2	
24 Hepar Sulphur.		
25 Hydrastus Canadensis.	Hydrastin	tr 0 p 2
26 Hamamelis Virginica.	Hamamelis Vir.	tr 0 p 3

27 Ipecacuanha.	Ipecac	tr 0 p 2 3
28 Laurocerasus.	Laurocerasus	p 3
29 Mercurius solubilis.	Merc.	tr 3
30 Mercurius corrosivus.	Mercurius cor.	tt 2 p 3
31 Macrotys Racemosa.	Macrotin,	tr 2
32 Nux Vomica.	Nux	p 3
33 Opium.	Opium	p 3
34 Phosphorus.	Phosphorus,	tr 2 p 3
35 Phosphoric acid.	Phos. acid,	tr 2 p 3
36 Podophyllum peltatum.	Podophyllin,	tt 1 p 3
37 Pulsatilla.	Pulsatilla	3
38 Rhus Toxicodendron.	Rhus Tox.	p 3
39 Secale cornutum.	Secale,	tr 1 p 3
40 Santonine.	Santonine,	tr 1
41 Spongia.	Spongia,	p 4
42 Tartar Emetic.	Tartar emetic	tr 2 p 3
43 Thuya.		
44 Veratrum alba.	Veratrum.	p 3

[Pg 5]

AN EPITOME

OF THE

HOMŒOPATHIC HEALING ART.

Introduction.

This work contains in a *condensed form* a very large portion of all that is practically useful in the treatment of the diseases ordinarily occurring in this country. The symptoms are given with sufficient minuteness and detail to enable any one of ordinary capacities of observation to distinguish the complaint; and the treatment is so *plainly* laid down, that no one need make a mistake. If strictly followed, [Pg 6] it will, in a very large proportion of cases, effect cures, even when administered by those unacquainted with the medical sciences generally. It has been written from necessity, to meet the demands of community for a more definite work in a concise form, that should contain remedies of the most reliable character, with such directions for their use as can be followed by the *traveler on his journey*, or by families at home, when no physician is at hand. It might seem to some preposterous to speak of a *demand* for another *domestic* Homœopathic Practice, when half a score or more of such works are now extant, some having come out within a very short time. The demand arises, not from the want of Books, but from the defects of those that exist. There is in most of them, too little point and definiteness in the prescriptions, and a kind of vague doubting recommendation noticeable to all, which carries the impression at once to every reader, of a want of *confidence* by the author in his own directions. [Pg 7]

Again, in some of the works there is too much confusion, the symptoms not being laid down with sufficient clearness to indicate the best remedy. Some of the works are unnecessarily large and cumbersome, while the real amount of valuable practical matter is comparatively meager, obliging the reader to pay for paper and binding without the contained value of his money. I do not claim entire perfection for this work, yet I do claim it to be several steps in advance of the books now extant.

This work is my own, being the result of my practical experience and observation. I have introduced several remedies that, though they are familiar to me, and have been used in my practice for many years, are, nevertheless, comparatively strange and new to most of the profession. Of some we have no extensive provings yet published, still the provings have been made, both upon the healthy and the sick. Their use, as directed in this work, is in strict accordance with their Homœopathic [Pg 8] relation to the symptoms for which they are prescribed.

Some may object to my practice of giving several remedies in alternation or rotation and in quick succession. To such I would say, When you try this mode of practice and on comparing it with the opposite one of giving only one remedy, and that at long intervals between the doses, find my mode to be less successful than yours, *then* it will be time for you to make your objections. *You* may rely upon the vague hypotheses of the books, and give your high dilutions singly, at long intervals, and let your patients die for want of *real* treatment, while I will use lower dilutions and give two or more remedies in quick succession and cure mine. I only speak what is in accordance with universal observation, where the two modes are compared on equal footing, when I affirm that, while the former *may* effect some cures, *most* of the recoveries under it, are spontaneous and unaided, the latter *does* cure; the disease being arrested by the medicine, and the proportion of unfavorable term [Pg 9] inations is much less under the latter than the former course. I know many learned and successful practitioners who have substituted low dilutions and the giving of several remedies in quick succession for the old mode of high attenuations and long intervals of single remedies, all of whom still adhere to the low, while I have yet to hear of the man who has gone *back* to high single remedies and long intervals. My reason then, for the course here laid down, is, that it will *cure* with more promptness and certainty. If others are so prejudiced as not to *try it*, they will still remain in ignorance of the *best practice*, and their patients will be the sufferers.

In reference to the fear that is expressed that if one medicine is given too soon after another, it will antidote the former, I have simply to say, I have no confidence in the hypothetic antidotal powers of the medicines one over another, as laid down in the books. It has not been verified by experience, and has no foundation in truth. It is true that one medicine will remove morbid symptoms that might be [Pg 10] produced by an overdose of another; but both being given in the ordinary medicinal doses, neither of them to such an extent as to produce sensible symptoms, if given alone, would not, if given in quick succession, prevent each other from acting to remove their own peculiar symptoms that exist in the system at the time. So if we have the symptoms that are found in two or more different remedies present in the same attack, as is often the ease, we may give these several remedies one after another, with confidence in their curative effects for the symptoms they represent.

This has been my practice, and it has been *eminently successful*, and therefore I commend it to others, treating with pity the infirmity of those who ignorantly condemn it, as "They know not what they do." [Pg 11]

ADMINISTRATION OF REMEDIES.

The remedies are either in the form of tinctures saturated, more or less dilute, in Pellets or Powders. The *Pellets* may be taken dry upon the tongue, allowed to dissolve and swallowed. The dose for an adult is from 4 to 7; for an infant, from birth to one year old, 1 to 3; from one to three years, 2 to 4; from three to ten years, 3 to 5 pellets; after ten, same as an adult. 15 or 20 pellets may be dissolved in a gill of water, and a tea-spoonful dose given at a time, being particular to stir it until all are perfectly dissolved, stirring it each dose.

Powders may be taken in the same manner, upon the tongue, a dose when dry, being about the same bulk as of the pellets as nearly as practicable. If put into water, to a gill of water add of the powder about what would lie on a three cent piece. If the liquid me [Pg 12] dicine is used, add 1 drop to a gill of water, and use tea-spoonful doses as above directed. The length of time between the doses should be, in Dysentery and Diarrhœa, regulated by the frequency of the discharges, giving a dose as often as the evacuations occur. In acute and violent diseases, the doses should be repeated oftener than in milder cases—about once an hour as a general rule is often enough, though in some cases they should be given in half an hour or oftener. In mild cases, once in two or three hours is often enough, and in chronic cases, once or twice a day.

Bathing.

The surface of the body should be kept clean, as far as possible, and to this end, in summer, should be well bathed at least once a day. In winter, though useful, it is not so indispensable; still no one should neglect the bath more than a week, and all ought to bathe at least twice a week, if not oftener, even in winter.

The bath should be of a temperature that is agreeable, and the room warm, especially for a feeble person. It should be so applied [Pg 13] as not to give a general chill, as such shocks are always hurtful.

The *teeth* should be kept clean and free from tartar. They should be cleaned every morning and after each meal. The feet, legs and arms should be warmly clothed, especially the *arms*, as an exposure of them to cold is liable to induce affections of the lungs, and to aggravate any existing disease of those organs.

By exposure of the feet and legs to cold, diseases and derangements of the female organs, even in young girls, are induced; and one prolific cause of female weakness is to be found in improper dressing of the feet and legs, while the *lung affections* of females, now so fearfully prevalent, are traceable in a great degree to the fashion that has prevailed for a few years, of exposing the arms to cold.

Diet.

The diet of the sick should he nutricious, but at all times simple, free from greasy substances, and from all stimulating condiments whatsoever, as well as from vinegar, or food in which vinegar is used. [Pg 14]

In short, let the food be nutritious, easily digested, small or moderate in quantity, and free from all "seasoning," except salt or sugar; and if salt is used at all, let the quantity be very small, much less than would be used in health.

Diarrhœa.

This disease consists in a looseness of the bowels, generally accompanied with pain in the abdomen, more or less severe. It sometimes occurs without pain, but is *then* attended with a sense of weakness, and a general feeling of uneasiness. It prevails mostly in the warm seasons, but may occur at any time. It is not usually considered a very dangerous affection, except during the prevalence of *Cholera*, or in children during hot weather.

TREATMENT.

Veratrum and *Phos. acid*, given alternately, at intervals, as frequently as the discharges from the bowels occur, will generally be sufficient. If there is nausea or vomiting, or cramping pains in the bowels, give *Ipecac* in alternation with one or both the former. If thirst and a burning of the stomach or bow [Pg 15] els exist, use *Arsenicum*. This last medicine may be given in alternation with either of the others, but is most frequently indicated in connection with *Veratrum*. The intervals between the doses should be regulated by the frequency of the evacuations in all cases, lengthening them as the evacuations become less frequent, until they cease. In *children*, where the discharges are greenish or slimy, and contain undigested food, give *Chamomilla* and *Ipecac* alternately, as above directed. If the discharges are dark, or yellow, with distress in the stomach, give *Podophyllin*. The dose is from 3 to 6 pellets. In all cases of diarrhœa, adults should abstain from all kinds of food until cured, if possible, and eat but little at first, when food is taken. Children should be fed carefully, and but a small quantity at a time, being particular both for adults and children to use as little *liquid* as possible; drink water in *small* quantities, not very cold. Avoid exercise, and lie on the back quietly, when that is practicable. In a large majority of cases, *Veratrum*, if given in the early stages of the disease, will arrest it at once, and in many [Pg 16] chronic diarrhœas of weeks or months standing, it is the surest remedy. In chronic diarrhœa of females, *Podophyllin* should be used in alternation with *Veratrum*.

Dysentery.

This disease is caused by inflammation of the mucous membrane of the colon and rectum, (the large intestine) generally confined to the lower part of the bowel. It is always painful. There is griping and straining in the lower part of the abdomen, and generally great bearing down when at stool, with a peculiar distress after the evacuation, called tormina.

The discharges often commence like a common diarrhœa, with copious liquid evacuations, but there is more or less griping pain, low down, from the beginning. The evacuations sooner or later become lessened, slimy or bloody, or both, the pain increasing accompanied with more or less fever, often quite severe. Sometimes the patient is costive, and has been so for several days, the dysentery coming on without being preceded by looseness. At others, especially in summer, when fevers are prevailing, the dysen [Pg 17] tery begins with a severe chill, followed by fever and the dysenteric symptoms above described.

TREATMENT.

If it begins with looseness without blood, give *Arsenicum* and *Veratrum* alternately, once an hour, or oftener if the evacuations are more frequent. If the discharges are bloody, use *Mercurius cor.* in place of the *Arsenicum.* If there is any sickness of the stomach, or the discharges are dark or yellow, use *Podophyllin* with *Mercurius cor.* If there are colic pains in the bowels, use *Colocynthis* alternately with the others, giving it between them. If the patient was costive previous to the attack, and the dysentery came on without much looseness, *Nux Vomica* should be given alternately with *Mercurius cor.* If the disease comes on with a chill, or a chill occurs at any time during the attack, followed by fever, *Aconite*, *Baptisia* and *Podophyllin* should be used in rotation half an hour apart until a free perspiration is produced, and the pain diminishes; or if bloody stools appear, use *Mer [Pg 18] curius cor*, with the *Aconite* and *Baptisia*. A large proportion of the dysenteries of hot weather in miasmatic regions, will be arrested in a few hours by these three or four remedies, especially if the patient keeps still, and generally even if he keeps about his business. In very bad cases, much benefit will be derived from injections of Gum Arabic water, or mucillage of Slippery Elm thrown into the bowel in quantities of a pint or more at a time, as warm as can possibly be endured. I have often relieved patients immediately with injections of a strong solution of Borax in Rice water, as hot as bearable. *Never apply cold water* to *any* inflamed surface, much less a *mucous* surface. All food should be withheld as far as practicable and not starve, until the symptoms abate.

Colic.

The symptoms of this are cramping pains in the abdomen, without fever or looseness of the bowels. The colic sometimes occurs after the cessation of a diarrhœa that had been induced by severe cathartics. The [Pg 19] pains are cutting and straining, drawing the bowels into knots, relieved temporarily by pressure.

TREATMENT.

For a male, *Nux Vom.*, and for a female, *Pulsatilla* will generally afford immediate relief. In children, especially, where diarrhœa exists, *Chamomilla* should be used. If it is the result of severe cathartics, or if there is a soreness or a bruised feeling, *Colocynth* is the remedy. Hot injections into the rectum, and large quantities of warm water taken into the stomach, will often *cure colic*.

Bilious Colic.

This disease, in addition to the symptoms of cutting, cramping pains in the bowels, as in common colic, has great distress in the stomach, with nausea and vomiting, the bowels being costive, the feet and hands cold, sometimes cold sweats occur. There is also considerable fever, and frequently headache is present. The substance vomited is at first dark bilious matter, but if the case continues a long time, stercoraceous (fecal) matter will be thrown up. [Pg 20]

TREATMENT.

Colocynth is the most important remedy, and should be given early and constantly. *Podophyllin* is next in importance, and it should be given in alternation with the former, the dose to be repeated as often as every half hour at first, and as the patient becomes easy, at longer intervals. In this, as in the former case, great benefit will be derived from large injections of quite warm water, and let it be taken into the stomach freely, as hot as can be safely swallowed. I have given a gallon of hot water in the course of two hours, to a patient suffering under this disease, the first half pint being rejected, but the balance remaining, perfect relief having been experienced. If fever continues after the colic and nausea cease, *Baptisia* and *Aconite* should be given alternately every hour until the fever subsides. If the patient is, and has been, for some time, costive, *Nux Vomica* should be given once in six or eight hours until the bowels move. Injections may also be used. [Pg 21]

Cholera Morbus.

This disease generally comes on at night, in hot weather, and is, in many cases, induced by over eating while the patient is suffering from diarrhœa and a deranged state of the liver. It is essentially of a bilious character. It sets in with great pain in the bowels, sickness at the stomach, and vomiting of large quantities of dark greenish bitter tasting substance. At first, the vomiting will seem to afford relief, but sooner or later the stomach and bowels cramp, and the cramping may extend to other parts of the body, the feet, hands, calves of the legs, and the arms, cold sweats come on, and death terminates his sufferings.

TREATMENT.

Ipecac and *Colocynthis* are to be given in alternation, and repeated as often as every 30 minutes, for the first three or four doses, then as the patient gets easier, at longer intervals. A dose every hour will suffice as soon as the symptoms begin to abate. The application of hot cloths or even mustard, over the abdomen, frequently palliates the sufferings, and does not interfere with the action of the me [Pg 22] dicines. Fever of a low typhoid type some times sets in after an attack of cholera morbus, and terminates fatally. This ought never to occur under Homœopathic treatment. For such fever give *Baptisia*, a dose every hour until the fever subsides, which will occur generally in six or eight hours; if not, and the patient complains of headache, or is delirious, or dizzy, or feels a fullness in the head, give *Macrotin* in alternation with the *Baptisia*. Keep the patient very quiet and free from noise, as far as possible. *Sleep* is a great restorer in any case, but particularly so in this.

FEVERS.

Intermittent Fever, Ague or Chill Fever.

This comes on with pains in the head and back, aching in the joints, yawning, followed by coldness of the hands and feet, blueness of the nails and skin of the hands, general chilliness, sometimes "shaking." This lasts from a few minutes in some cases, to several hours in others. The chill is followed by a fever, which is generally severe and long continued, in proportion to the length and [Pg 23] severity of the chill. The fever is followed by free perspiration, when it subsides and leaves the patient in a comfortable condition. This state is called the *Intermission*. This continues from a few hours to twenty-four, or longer, when another chill comes on followed by fever and sweats as before. During the chill and fever, the patient often suffers great pain, and is sometimes delirious. Young children frequently have convulsions when the chill sets in. *These* convulsions of children, though alarming, are not often dangerous.

TREATMENT.

As soon as the first symptoms of the chills appear, such as the headache, pain in the back and bones, coldness of the hands, nose and ears, give *Aconite* and *Baptisia* alternately, giving the first three doses every ten minutes, the next three doses every fifteen minutes, and then once in half an hour until the patient begins to sweat freely, when the medicines should be discontinued. If there is nausea or vomiting present, let the patient have lukewarm water freely in large draughts, until he vomits it up several times. [Pg 24] As soon as the sweating commences, give *Arsenicum* and *Macrotin* alternately every hour during the intermission, except during sleeping time. On return of the chill, should it appear a second time, use the *Aconite* and *Baptisia* as before, and follow them with *Arsenicum* and *Nux Vom.* every two hours. This course of treatment will cure a majority of cases, but some require *Cinchonia*. That Cinchonia is a specific for intermittent fevers in many of their forms, no one will deny. It is the Homœopathic remedy for many cases, and should be prescribed. The injurious effects that are often attributed to Quinine, are, I have no doubt, attributable not to that remedy, but to the *drugs* that are used prior to giving the *Chinium Sul*. I have used it in more than two thousand cases, and have never been able to see any evil consequences follow its *proper* use. It should be given *from the beginning of the chill to the end* of the paroxysm, and continued during the whole time of the intermission: *i. e.* until the time arrives for the next chill, *time* being important in the use of this remedy. Use the first decimal tritu [Pg 25] ration, and give grain doses (equal to 1-10th of a grain of the drug) every half hour till the time the next chill would occur, if it pursued its regular course, allowing the patient six or seven hours time in each twenty-four, for sleep. [1] Though from two to four grains of the pure *Chinium Sulphuricum* is all the patient would get, very few cases that do not yield to a course of the former treatment here recommended, will have the third paroxysm after this *China* treatment is commenced and pursued as here directed. For children the dose may be one-half or one-fourth that of the adults. If a trituration [Pg 26] of the medicine cannot be got conveniently, four grains of the *Quinine* may be put into a four ounce vial of water, shaken well every time, and a teaspoonful taken at a dose. Abstinence from food as far as practicable, and quiet is of much importance in this disease, but the patient may use water freely.

In some cases, the chill is irregular and indistinct, the patient is thirsty during the chill, and the cold stage is long in proportion to the length of the fever, the surface pale and more or less bloated. *Arsenicum* is the remedy, and should be given from the commencement of the chill, and every hour until the fever subsides, then every three hours during the intermission. In chronic cases, where the patient has been drugged with mercurials and cathartics, together with larger doses of Quinine, and is still suffering under the disease, *Pulsatilla* and *Macrotin* in alternation, will, in nearly every case, effect a cure.

Bilious Fever.

This fever may be either intermittent, remitting, or continued, and typhoid. It is distinguished from common intermittent, by [Pg 27] the great derangement of the stomach, as nausea and vomiting of bilious matter, yellow coated tongue, bitter taste in the mouth, foul breath, loss of appetite, high colored urine, and frequently distress and fullness in the right side, (though this last is not in every case present,) the skin and white of the eyes soon become yellowish, the chills are often imperfect, the fever being disproportionably long.

TREATMENT.

Podophyllin and *Merc.* should be given in ease of intermittents of this character, during the paroxysm, and in rotation with the other remedies for intermittents, giving a dose every three hours during the intermission. It is well also to continue these remedies night and morning, alternately, for a week or so, after the cessation of the chills and fever, or until all bilious appearances cease.

A Remitting Fever is one that goes nearly off, but not so entirely as an intermittent, returning again by a paroxysm of chill more or less distinct, sometimes hardly [Pg 28] perceptible, and an increase of the fever following, from day to day, until arrested.

Continued Fevers are generally of a Bilious character, except in winter, when they are more or less connected with irritation of the lungs, or with Rheumatic affections, when they are termed Catarrhal or Rheumatic Fevers. If the bilious symptoms prevail, give *Aconite* and *Baptisia* during the chills and high febrile stage, at intervals of an hour, and during the declining stage of the fever, give *Podophyllin* and *Mercurius* until a perfect intermission is produced, when the same treatment should be adopted as in intermittents. But should it take the form of

Catarrhal Fever,

the head being "stuffed up," pain in the head, the lungs oppressed, cough and sneezing, the eyes and nose suffused with increased secretion of tears and mucus, pain in the back or loins, almost constant chilly sensations, use in rotation *Baptisia*, *Copaiva* and *Phosphorus*, giving a dose every hour until the fever begins to abate and perspiration comes [Pg 29] on, then leave off the *Baptisia*, and give in its stead *Macrotin*, lengthening the interval between the remedies to two hours or longer.

For the *chronic cough* that sometimes follows catarrhal fever, *Copaiva*, *Macrotin* and *Phosphorus* should be used morning, noon and night, in the order here named. Should the fever be a

Rheumatic Fever,

(*Rheumatism*,) the patient complaining of soreness of the muscles, of the chest, back and limbs, with or without lameness of the joints, *Aconite*, *Macrotin* and *Nux Vom.* are the remedies for a male patient, and the two former, with *Pulsatilla*, for a female, (or for a *male*, of light hair, delicate skin, feminine voice and mild temper,) to be used in rotation one hour apart. These remedies are to be taken in a severe acute case, every half hour until the symptoms begin to abate; then every hour or two hours as the case progresses. *Baths* properly administered, are of great importance in all forms of fever. The surface of the patient should be washed and thoroughly *rubbed* in water quite warm, into [Pg 30] which a sufficiency of the ley of wood ashes has been put to make it feel quite slippery. This should be done twice daily in all fevers. But in

Rheumatism,

In addition to the medicines directed under the head of *Rheumatic Fever*, the most decided benefit can be derived from *Alcoholic Vapor Baths*, which, while they do not in the least interfere with the action of the medicines, tend greatly to mitigate the pains, and produce an equal state of the circulation by stimulating the surface; abridging in many cases, the disease one-half the time it would run under the long interval treatment alone. This is to be applied by filling a tea cup with alcohol, placed in a saucer of water to insure against danger from an overflow while burning. Place both under a solid wood bottom chair, elevated about the thickness of a brick under each post, strip the patient naked, and after giving him the alkaline bath, and rubbing his surface dry, place him upon the chair, enveloping him completely, except his head, with a woollen sheet or blanket, [Pg 31] (as there is no danger of the wool taking fire,) letting the blanket enclose also the chair and come down to the floor. Then set fire to the alcohol, and if the heat is too great, raise the edge of the blanket and let it become reduced. Continue this until he sweats freely, or becomes too much fatigued to sit longer. Let the patient often drink freely of cold water, during the process. Remove him from the chair to his bed and cover him warmly. It is well to place the feet in hot water during this process. This is a delightful operation for a rheumatic patient, and no one will object to a repetition of it. Whatever Physicians may think or say of this operation, I *know* it is a most potent agent for the *cure* of *inflammatory* rheumatism, and is a valuable agent in the chronic form of this disease.

Typhoid Fever.

This is a dangerous, and with the ordinary allopathic treatment, a very fatal disease. It generally comes on insidiously, the patient feeling a dull head ache, more or less pain in his joints, back and shoulders, with loss [Pg 32] of appetite, restless and disturbed sleep, slight chilly sensations, with a little fever, dry skin, and a general languid feeling. These symptoms continue from four or five days in some cases, to two or three weeks in others, gradually getting worse until the patient is prostrated, or if he takes no drugs, and keeps still, avoiding food as far as practicable, he may escape prostration, and after lingering for eight or ten days, and sometimes longer, just on the point of prostration, he begins slowly to get better, and recovers about as slowly and imperceptibly as he grew sick. This is in accordance with observation of cases under my own eye, and I have no doubt those cases of spontaneous recovery, had they taken a single dose of active cathartic medicine or any of the active drugs, they would have been immediately laid upon a bed of sickness from which a recovery would have been extremely doubtful. I believe that two-thirds of the deaths from typhoid fever are the direct results of medication, and that those who recover, do so in spite of the cathartics and the active drugs when such are used. Some cases, however, [Pg 33] will not thus spontaneously recover, and require proper treatment; and it is safest to treat all cases, at as early a day as possible. Some cases come on more rapidly and run into the prostrating or critical stage, in a very few days. Delirium is a symptom that comes on early in these cases. When the disease is fully established, and even sometimes in the early stage, diarrhœa sets in and runs the patient down rapidly.

TREATMENT.

In the early stage, that which might be called premonitory, while the patient is yet able to be about his business, but is complaining of the symptoms above named, he should, as far as possible, abstain from exercise and food, and take of *Baptisia* and *Phosphorus* alternately, a dose once in three hours. These will almost invariably produce amendment in a few days, and as soon as he improves *any*, leave off the medicines. Should there be diarrhœa present, use *Phos.*

acid instead of Phosphorus. If the patient is delirious or has fullness and redness of the face, the eyes red, and headache, give *Bella [Pg 34] donna* in rotation with the other two. For the foul breath that comes on, use *Mercurius cor.*, especially if the diarrhœa assumes a reddish tinge, like beef brine. Should the fever at any time rise high, the pulse being full and hard, give *Aconite*, but it rarely happens that Aconite is useful in the later stage. If the patient complains of pains in the back, and fullness of the head, give *Macrotin*. This is particularly useful for persons who have rheumatic pains in the limbs or back, during the fever. If the evacuations from the bowels are dark, or yellow and consistent, or there is bilious vomiting, *Podophyllin* is the remedy. From some cause or other, to me wholly unaccountable, the writers generally have laid down *Rhus* and *Bryonia* as *the* remedies in typhoid fever. I must confess I have no confidence in them for this fever as it prevails, and has for several years past, in this country. They have proved a failure, and I discard them altogether, as I am confident, from thorough trial, we have much more reliable remedies as a substitute for Rhus in the *Podophyllin*, and for Bryonia in the *Macrotin*. In the [Pg 35] early stage, or at any time to arrest febrile and inflammatory symptoms, the *Baptisia* is much more potent than Aconite, its symptoms corresponding peculiarly with typhoid fever. If the discharges become slimy or bloody, give *Leptandrin* and *Nit. acid*. It is important to bathe in this disease.

Scarlet Fever.—Scarlatina.

This fever assumes two principal forms: Simple or mild, and Malignant. In the *Simple form*, there is great heat of the surface, extremely quick and frequent pulse, headache, and some sense of pain and soreness in the throat. After a day or two, there appears upon the surface, bright scarlet patches, in some cases extending over the whole limbs, the skin smooth and shining, and somewhat bloated or swollen; upon pressure with the finger, a white spot is seen, which soon disappears on removal of the pressure. As the disease subsides, the cuticle comes off (*desquamates*) in patches. In the simple form of this disease, the throat, though often more or less sore, does not ulcerate. In some cases, notwithstanding the fever is high, the pulse frequent, and the [Pg 36] throat sore, there may be no external redness, but the mouth and tongue will have a scarlet hue, indicating the existence of disease more dangerous than when it appears externally. *In the malignant form*, the same symptoms are present, the patient suffers more pain in the head; the back and throat, root of the tongue, tonsils and soft palate become ulcerated, turn black, and sometimes gangrenous, proving fatal in a few days, or slough out in large portions, the ulcers destroying the parts extensively. The breath becomes foul and fetid, and the effluvia from the ulcerated surface, is very sickening to the patient and all around him. This disease rarely attacks adults, but occasionally, and for the last six or eight months, in one region where I am acquainted, where Scarlatina of a malignant type has prevailed among children, adults have been affected with an epidemic soreness of the mouth and throat, strongly resembling the worst form of the *angina* in malignant Scarlatina, together with a low typhoid form of fever. [Pg 37]

TREATMENT.

In simple scarlatina, all that is necessary is to keep the child quiet, in a room of uniform temperature, as far as practicable; let it drink cold water only, and give *Aconite, Belladonna* and *Pulsatilla* in rotation, a dose every hour until the fever subsides. If any soreness of the throat remains, give a few doses of *Mercurius*. If the fever subsides, and the soreness remain, *Hydrastin* or *Eupatorium arom.* will soon complete the cure. In the *malignant* form, with ulcerated, dark colored, or red and purulent throat, and typhoid form of fever, give *Aconite* and *Belladonna* in alternation, every hour, and, at the same time, gargle the throat freely with *Hydrastin*. Some of the tincture may be put in water, about in the proportion of ten drops to a teaspoonful, or a warm infusion of the crude medicine may be used. This can be applied with a camel's hair pencil, or a swab, to the parts affected, once in two hours, and will soon bring about such a state as will result in speedy recovery. After the active fever has subsided, the *Aconite* and *Bell.* may be discontinued, and *Eupatorium* [Pg 38] *arom.* used instead, once in three hours until convalescence is complete.

I would remark that, with these remedies applied as here recommended, my brother, Dr. G. S. Hill, of Erie County, Ohio, has, during the last four months, treated a large number of those malignant sore-throats, (the "Black tongue Erysipelas,") and been universally successful, relieving them in a few hours, when the symptoms were of the most alarming character, and the disease in some cases, so far advanced that the patients were considered by their friends and attendants, "at the point of death."

The *Hydrastin* is a most potent remedy in putrid ulcerations of the mucous surfaces, and much the same may be said of *Eupatorium aromaticum*.

Yellow Fever.

[As I have never practiced farther South than Cincinnati, and have seen but few cases of this disease, my experience with it has not been sufficient to be relied upon as authority. Therefore, I shall give a brief description of the disease, with the proper [Pg 39] and *successful treatment*, furnished me by A. H. Burrett, M. D., of New Orleans, who is not only a Physician of more than ordinary learning and skill in his profession generally, but is one who has spent his time in New Orleans among the sick of Yellow Fever, through three of the most fatal epidemics that ever scourged any city. He is a man for the times, a man of resources, who draws useful lessons from experience and observation. Hence he has been able to select such remedies as have enabled him to cope most successfully with the pestilence, saving nearly all his patients, while, under other treatment, a majority have died. I therefore, attach great value to his treatment, and recommend its adoption with the most implicit confidence.]

When this Fever prevails as an epidemic, as it usually does, in the southern part of the United States, it is a disease of the most malignant character. The proportion of *fatal* cases under the Allopathic course of treatment, has been equal to, and, in some places, as in New Orleans, and some Towns [Pg 40] in Virginia, has exceeded that of *Asiatic* Cholera. It is almost entirely confined to Southern regions, and only prevails in hot weather, after the continuance of extreme heat for some weeks.

It usually begins with premonitory symptoms somewhat like those of ordinary fever, but with this difference: the patient, instead of losing his appetite, has often a morbidly increased desire for food. He complains of severe pains in the back, and more or less headache. Both the head and backache are of a peculiar character: the pains resembling rheumatic pains, the head feeling full and too large, the eyes early turn red, almost bloodshot and watery, a chill comes on, which may be distinct and quite severe, lasting for an hour or more, or, it may be slight, and hardly perceptible. The chill is followed by high fever, the pain in the head and back increasing, the eyes becoming more red and suffused, the forehead and face extremely red and hot, and the heat of the whole surface very great, the carotids beat violently, the pulse very frequent, and usually, at first, full and strong, though some [Pg 41] times it is feeble from the beginning. However the pulse may be in the beginning, it very soon becomes small, but continues to be frequent. The tongue is at first covered with a white paste-like coating, which afterwards gives place to redness of the edges and tip, with a dark or yellow streak in the center. The stomach is very irritable, rejecting every kind of food, and all drinks, except, perhaps, a few drops of ice water. There is a peculiar distressed feeling in the stomach, often a burning sensation, so that, if suffered to do so, he would take large quantities of ice or water. One remarkable feature of the cases noticed in the epidemic, as it existed in New Orleans the past season, was, that the patients had a great desire for food, notwithstanding the nausea and distress at the stomach.

Sooner or later, varying from a few hours to several days, in the ordinary course of the disease, the fever subsides. From this time the patient may recover without any further symptoms, but this is, by no means, the usual result. If the subsidence of the fever is accompanied by natural pulse, a free, but [Pg 42] not profuse or prostrating perspiration, a genial warmth of the surface, natural appearance of the countenance, eyes, and tongue, with little or no soreness on pressure over the stomach, we may safely look for a speedy recovery. But if, on the contrary, the eyes, face, and tongue, become yellow, or orange-colored, the epigastrium is tender to pressure, the urine has a yellow tinge, the pulse becomes unnaturally slow, with the least degree of mental stupor, we have reason to know, full well, that the lull of the fever is only the calm preceding a more destructive storm. The fever has subsided, only because exhausted nature could re-act no longer. It may be in a few hours, or not until twelve or twenty-four have elapsed, the pulse becomes quickened, even to the frequency of 120 to 140 in a minute, but very feeble, the extremities of the fingers and toes turn purple or dark, the tongue becomes brown and dry, or is clean, red, and cracked, sordes may be on the teeth, the stomach become more irritable, nausea and vomiting are extreme, the substances vomited being, at first, reddish, afterwards watery, containing floculæ, like [Pg 43] soot, or coffee grounds; the breath becomes foul, and the whole surface emits a sickening odor.

The pulse becomes very small, though the carotid and temporal arteries beat violently. The urine fails to be secreted, and later, blood is discharged from the mucous surfaces, involuntary discharges from the bowels, clammy sweats; and death follows.

The disease runs its course in from three to seven days, sometimes proves fatal in less than a day, and at others, assumes a typhoid form, and runs for weeks. Occasionally it sets in without any of the premonitory symptoms, the chill being first, the fever following, succeeded immediately by the black vomit, going through all the stages in a single day, or two days.

Again, it sometimes begins with the black vomit, the patient being immediately prostrated. In all cases, however it may begin, the peculiar head-ache and back-ache as described in the beginning, as well as the extreme heat of the head and face, redness of the eyes, the gnawing sensation at the stomach, and peculiar nausea are present. These seem to be characteristic symptoms that [Pg 44] mark the Yellow Fever, and those which should guide in the search for the proper remedies.

TREATMENT.

The remedies that proved successful in arresting the disease during the early or forming stage, before the chill or fever had set in, while the symptoms were pain, fullness, and throbbing of the head, with more or less dizziness, rheumatic pains in the back, and redness of the eyes, were *Aconite* and *Bell.*, at low attenuations, once in two to four hours, according to the violence of the symptoms. For the fullness of the head, pressing outwards, as though it would split, with pains of a rheumatic character, *Macrotin* 1st, given in one grain doses, every hour or two hours, proved specific.

These three remedies, *Aconite, Bell.* and *Macrotin*, would, in nearly all cases, arrest the disease in the forming stage, so that no chill or fever would occur, or, if fever did come on after this treatment, it was mild.

When the fever sets in, and the pain in the head and back increases, the eyes, forehead and face are extremely red, or purple [Pg 45] and hot, the pulse frequent and full, the tongue coated white, *Aconite*, *Belladonna* and *Macrotin* are still to be relied upon, but they should be given every half hour, in rotation, at low attenuations. If the tongue is red, in the early stage, use *Bryonia* in place of the *Belladonna*. In a later stage, when sickness or distress at the stomach had become prominent, with the quick pulse, and hot skin, *Ipecac* and *Aconite*, both at the 1st attenuation, a dose given every half hour alternately, generally arrested the symptoms, and brought on perspiration of a healthful character, followed by subsidence of the fever and convalescence. Sponge baths, with half an ounce of *Tr. Ipecac* in two quarts of tepid water, applied to the whole surface freely, under the bed clothes, so as not to expose him to the air, contributed much towards bringing on perspiration and subduing the fever, as well as allaying the nausea.

When called to patients in the stage of *Black Vomit*, whether that came on as an early symptom, or at a later stage, *Nit. acid*, *Veratrum virid.* and *Baptisia*, all at the first dilution, were administered every hour, in [Pg 46] rotation, with great success, the symptoms yielding in a few hours. For the great oppression, as of a load, in the stomach, without vomiting, *Nux* was found sufficient. In the later stage, when there seemed to be no secretion of urine, *Canabis* and *Apis mel.*, gave relief.

The remedies most successful for the cases that assumed a typhoid character, with dry, cracked tongue, sordes on the teeth, and low sluggish pulse, were *Baptisia* and *Bryonia*, given every two hours, alternately. *Nitric acid* given internally and injected into the rectum, when bloody discharges appear, is generally quite successful.

Good nursing is of the utmost importance, and the patient should be visited frequently by his Physician, as great changes may occur in a short time. Three times a day is none too often to see the patient. As soon as the fever comes on, the patient should be stripped of his clothes, and dressed in such garments as he is to wear in bed through the attack. He should be put to bed and lightly covered, but have sufficient to protect him from any sudden changes in the atmosphere, and the [Pg 47] room should be well ventilated all the time. The baths should always be applied under the bed clothes.

The diet should be very spare and light, after the fever subsides, and while the fever exists no food should be taken. Thin gruel, in teaspoonful doses, once in half an hour, is best. After a day or two, the juice of beef steak may be given in small quantities but give none of the meat. No "hearty food" should be allowed for eight or ten days after recovery. A relapse is most surely fatal.

As *Prophylactics* (*preventives*) of the fever, *Macrotin*, *Bell.* and *Aconite* should be taken, a dose every eight to twelve hours, by every one that is exposed. These will, no doubt, often prevent an attack, and if they do not, they will so modify it, that it will be very mild, of short duration, and very easily arrested.

Pregnant females, and young children were sure to die if attacked, when treated by the Allopathic medication; but, by the use of these remedies as *preventives*, their attacks were rendered so mild as to be amenable to remedies, and all recovered. [Pg 48]

Pleurisy—Pleuritis.

This is inflammation of the Pleura of one or both lungs, generally confined to one side. It is known by sharp pain in the side of the chest, increased by taking a long breath, or coughing, or by pressing between the ribs. The cough is dry and painful, the patient makes an effort to suppress it, from the pain it gives him; the fever is of a high grade, the pulse full, hard and frequent, with more or less pain in the head.

TREATMENT.

Aconite is a sovereign remedy. It should be given at intervals proportionate to the severity of the disease, once in half an hour, for about three doses, then every hour until the patient is easy and perspires freely. This is the course I have generally pursued, and scarce ever failed of relieving in a few hours. Other means may often be used with advantage at the same time, and not interfere with the action of the medicine. Put the feet and *hands* into water as hot as it can be endured, and apply to the affected side very hot cloths, hot bags of salt, or mustard. There is no [Pg 49] harm in this, and it relieves the pain. Let the patient drink freely of *hot* water, into which you may put milk and sugar to render it palatable. If the case seems to linger, and perspiration is tardy in appearing, give, in alternation with *Aconite*, *Eupatorium arom.* This will soon relieve.

Inflammation of the Lungs—Pneumonia.

This disease is often connected with Pleurisy, and consists of inflammation of the substance of the lungs. As in the former case, it may attack only one, but may exist in both sides at the same time. If the pleura is also affected, there will be all the symptoms of pleurisy, together with those peculiar to inflammation of the lungs proper. They are, pain in the lungs, oppressed breathing, cough, causing great distress on account of the soreness of the affected parts: at first, expectoration from the lungs is nearly wanting, the cough being dry, but after a time, there is a rattling sound on coughing, and more or less mucous substance is with difficulty raised. This is, at first, white or brownish, but soon becomes reddish and frothy, tinged with [Pg 50] blood. The patient lies on the affected side, and cannot rest on the sound side. The pulse is full, hard and frequent, the fever high, pain in the head, and sometimes delirium. If the disease is not arrested, the patient generally dies from suffocation, by the lungs filling up, hepatized, or abscess and ulceration come on, and then what is called "quick Consumption" carries him off.

TREATMENT.

In the early stage, *Aconite* and *Phosphorus* should be used at intervals of from half an hour to one hour, in alternation, until the fever abates, and the oppression in the chest is relieved. If, however, there is bloody expectoration, *Bryonia* may be used in place *of Phosphorus*, though I prefer to use it in rotation with the two others. These will soon, in all ordinary cases, subdue the most distressing symptoms, and effect a perfect cure in a day or two. *Belladonna* should be used, when there is much delirium, or great pain in the head. Occasionally, the cough from the beginning, is apparently loose; there being a rattling sound, but the expectoration [Pg 51] is difficult, the fever high, with some chilly sensations, or at least, coldness of the knees, feet and hands, a white or brownish fur upon the tongue, and pain in the bowels, For such symptoms, especially with the pain in the bowels, as though a diarrhœa would come on, give *Tartar emet.* It is often one of the best remedies in this disease, affording relief when others have failed.

After subduing the high febrile symptoms, if there remains cough, indicating much irritation, or inflammation of the lungs, *Macrotin* should be used in place of Aconite, with *Phosphorus* and *Copaiva*, the three in rotation, two hours between doses.

Acute Bronchitis,

Inflammation of the Bronchial Tubes.

This is attended with distressing cough, profuse expectoration, oppressed breathing, pain in the forehead, and general catarrhal symptoms. *Baptisia*, *Copaiva* and *Eupatorium arom.* given every hour, in rotation, will, in general, relieve from the acute affection in a short time; but the [Pg 52]

Chronic Bronchitis

requires the use of *Copaiva*, *Macrotin* and *Arum triphyllum*, to be taken morning, noon, and night, in the order named; or, if the cough be severe, they should be used every three hours. These will be sufficient to effect a cure.

Coughs

Generally, unless they arise from consumption, yield readily to the alternate use of *Copaiva*, *Phosphorus* and *Macrotin*, a dose given once in from three to six hours. If, however, there is soreness of the throat, redness and soreness of the tonsils, palate, and fauces, or soreness of the larynx, with hoarseness, *Arum triphyllum* and *Hydrastus Can.* are the surest remedies. They rarely ever fail of effecting a complete cure in a few days. They should be used three or four times a day. They may be used with the other medicines recommended for coughs. In acute

Sore Throat,

arising from sudden cold, *Arum triphyllum* and *Eupatorium aromaticum* are the reme [Pg 53] dies to be relied upon. If the tonsils seem to be mainly involved, constituting

Quinsy — Tonsilitis,

Belladonna and *Aconite* should be given, while there is high fever, then substitute for them, *Arum tri.* and *Phosphorus*; or, these may be used in rotation with the former, a dose every hour or oftener.

Inflammation of the Bowels. — Enteritis.

This consists in inflammation of the muscular and peritoneal coats of the intestines, sometimes also involving the mucous coat.

The pain in the abdomen is constant, intense and burning in its character, felt most at the navel; the abdomen is extremely tender to pressure, and often bloated or tympanetic.

Thirst is intense, but cold drinks distress and vomit the patient. The pulse is small, feeble and frequent, and the bowels costive. This is a very dangerous disease. It is sometimes connected with inflammation of the stomach, then called gastro-enteritis. The tongue is then red and pointed, the nausea and vomiting are more violent and constant, the thirst burning and insatiable. [Pg 54]

TREATMENT.

The same medicines are applicable to both *Gastritis* and *Enteritis*.

Aconite, *Arsenicum* and *Baptisia* should be used one following the other every half hour until the symptoms begin to subside, then let the intervals be lengthened.

In addition to these remedies, I allow the patient to drink often and freely of hot water, as hot as can be swallowed, and though it is at first almost instantly rejected by the stomach, by repeating it in a few minutes in moderate quantities, it gives relief and will soon so allay the irritation as to remain. In some cases the vomiting is severe, the bowels are loose, and pain burning. For such, *Tart. Emet.* is the proper remedy. Cold drinks should not be taken.

Cloths wet in cold water, ice water if it is at hand, and wrung out so as not to drip, should be laid over the whole abdomen and instantly covered with two or three thicknesses of warm dry flannel, and the patient's feet kept warm. This may be considered harsh treatment, but there is no danger in it; on the contrary I have, in the worst and [Pg 55] most alarming cases of *gastritis* and *peritonitis*, made such applications, and in less than an hour have seen my patient easy and beginning to perspire freely, all danger having passed. It always affords more or less relief and is never attended with danger. Covering the wet cloths immediately with plenty of dry ones is very essential.

After the acute inflammation has subsided, it is well to have the bowels moved, but don't give drastic cathartics. *Nux Vomica* given at night and repeated morning and noon, will generally serve to cause an evacuation. Injections may be used.

Croup.

This is a disease of children. Comes on in consequence of a sudden cold. Children suffering from Hooping Cough are more subject to it. The cough is of a peculiar whistling kind, like the crowing of a young chicken, with rattling in the throat and difficult breathing, fever is present, and often very violent. It is properly an inflammation of the Larynx, but the inflammation may also exist in the Pharynx, the tonsils may be involved, and it may extend to the trachia, [Pg 56] (wind pipe). A false membrane forms in the larynx if the disease is not arrested, and so obstructs the breathing as to cause death from suffocation.

TREATMENT.

Give at first *Aconite*, *Phosphoric Acid*, and *Spongia*, giving them in the order here named once in ten minutes in a very violent case, and as the patient improves at intervals of half an hour, and then an hour.

Should the fever subside, and still the tightness in the throat and cough continue to be troublesome, give *Ipecac* in place of Aconite. And when the cough seems to be deep seated use *Bryonia* instead of spongia.

The patient should be kept in a warm room, and free from exposure to currents of cold air. The application of a cloth wrung out of cold or ice water to the throat, covered immediately with dry warm flannels so as to exclude the air from the wet cloth, will often exert a decidedly beneficial effect, and there is no danger if managed as here directed. The feet should be kept warm and the head cool, but *don't* put *cold* water on a child's head. [Pg 57]

Asthma.

If an attack comes on from sudden cold, take *Aconite* and *Ipecac* every hour for a day, and if any symptoms remain, in place of the Aconite use *Copaiva*, *Arsenicum* and *Phos. Acid* with the *Ipecac*, giving them in rotation, a dose every hour.

In *Chronic Asthma*, where the patient is liable to an attack at any time, great benefit will be derived from taking these four in rotation about two hours apart for a day or two, at any time when symptoms of an attack begin to appear.

I have recently succeeded in alleviating several bad cases, at once, by these four remedies in succession as here recommended, on whom (some of them) I had at various times tried all of them, as well as other medicines, singly at longer intervals, as directed in the Books, without any decided benefit. After trying these in succession, as here directed, I found no trouble in arresting the paroxysm in a few hours, and I am strong in the faith that with some, at least, I have effected *cures*. It is worth much to *arrest* the *paroxysm* if no more. [Pg 58]

Hooping Cough.

According to my experience, though this disease may not be entirely arrested in its course, and not generally much abridged in its duration, still the use of appropriate medicines will greatly modify it, and render it a comparatively trifling affection.

In treatment, give at the commencement of the attack *Bell.* and *Phos. acid* alternately every twelve hours for a week, then once in six hours, and if the child should take cold so as to bring on fever, give one every hour. Continue these, as above directed, for the first two or three weeks, then, in their stead, after the cough becomes loose, and the patient vomits easily, give *Copaiva and Ipecac* in the same manner as directed, for the two former remedies.

Dyspepsia.

This term is applied so loosely and so indiscriminately to all chronic derangements of the stomach, that it is difficult to define it. I shall therefore point out some of the more common ailments of the stomach and their proper remedies. [Pg 59]

For sour eructations with hot, burning, scalding fluid rising up in the throat, with or without food, give *Phos. acid and Pulsatilla* in alternation every half hour, until the stomach is easy. For a feeling of weight and pain in the stomach, with dull pain in the head, with or without dizziness, give *Nux. Vom.* every hour until it relieves. If there is a *burning* feeling in the stomach as well as the heavy load, *without* eructations and rising of fluid, *Arsenicum* should be alternated with the *Nux. Vom.*, at intervals of two hours. There are persons who, from imprudence in eating or drinking or both, or which is more frequent, from *harsh drug medication*, have so enfeebled their stomachs, that, though by care in selecting their food, and prudence in taking it, they may suffer but little, are, nevertheless, when from home or on special occasions, liable to overeat or take the wrong kind of food, from which unfortunate circumstance they are made to suffer the most tormenting and intolerable distress in the stomach and bowels, which may last, more or less severe, for several days. Soon after the unfortunate [Pg 60] meal, perhaps the next morning, or, it may be, in a few hours, the stomach begins to bloat, by accumulating gas within, which is belched up every few minutes in large quantities; the stomach and bowels are racked with the most torturing pains; cold sweat stands on the brow, and he is the very picture of misery. Thus he may roll and tumble all night, and remain in misery the next day and several days longer, before the food will digest. It often passes from the stomach without digestion, and on its way through the bowels inflicts constant pain. If he does not take some emetic substance, he is not apt to vomit, his stomach cramping so as to prevent it.

I have here described one of the bad cases, but bad as it is they are by no means *very* rare. There are such cases in abundance, of all grades from the one here described down to a slight derangement. They all require a similar course of *treatment*.

It is useful for such patients to take at once large quantities of lukewarm water, and repeat the draught every ten to fifteen minutes, until free and thorough vomiting is induced, [Pg 61] so as to throw off all the food from the stomach.

But even this does not often cure these bad cases. If it did, it is not always convenient to do it. The medicine that is quite certain to afford relief at once is *Podophyllin*. Let it be given, and the dose repeated in an hour. A third dose is rarely necessary. After relief from this attack, the medicine should be taken night and morning for a month or more until the stomach is restored. In the meantime care should be taken not to overload the stomach.

Constipation.

The medicine for this affection is *Nux vom.*, to be taken at night on retiring. If there is fulness and pain in the head from costiveness, *Bell.* should be used in the morning, and at noon. Let the patient contract a habit of drinking *cold water* freely on rising in the morning, at least half an hour before eating. The patient *should not take physic*.

For constipation of children, *Nux* and *Bryonia* are to be given Nux at night and Bryonia in the morning. *Opium* is useful. [Pg 62]

Much needless alarm is often felt by persons on account of a costive state of the bowels. If no pain is felt from it, there is no cause for alarm.

"Heartburn."

This peculiar burning and distressed feeling at the stomach depends on imperfect digestion, but is *not* ordinarily, as is generally supposed, connected with a sour or acid state of the fluids in the stomach. The condition of the fluids is alkaline, in most cases, though it is sometimes acid. If it depends upon biliary derangement, *Nux Vomica* and *Podophyllin* are the remedies for a male; *Pulsatilla* and *Podophyllin* for a female.

Erysipelas.

This is a disease of the skin, producing redness, burning and itching pains, appearing in patches, in adults, most apt to appear about the head and face, but in children, upon the limbs, or in very young children, beginning at the umbilicus. It sometimes begins at one point, and continues to spread for a time, then suddenly disappears, and reappears at some other point. [Pg 63]

Simple Erysipelas only affects the surface, with redness and smarting. *Vessicular*, produces vessicular eruption, or blisters filled with a limpid fluid, somewhat like the blisters from a burn.

The *Phlegmonous Erysipelas* affects the whole thickness of the skin and cellular tissues beneath it, producing swelling, and not unfrequently, resulting in suppuration, ulceration or gangrene and sloughing of the parts. It is a dangerous disease, especially when on the head.

TREATMENT.

For the simple kind, *Bell.* is all that will be needed, unless there should be considerable fever, when *Aconite* should be alternated with the *Bell.* For the *vessicular* kind, where there are blisters, *Rhus tox.* should be used with *Bell*. For the *Phlegmonous*, with deep seated swellings, *Apis mel* is the most important remedy. I prefer to use three of these remedies, giving them in rotation, beginning with the *Bell.*, followed with *Rhus*, and then by *Apis mel.* giving them one hour apart. In a mild case, or after the patient begins to recover, give them at longer inter [Pg 64] vals. The *Apis* alone will often be sufficient. During the whole time, the affected parts should be kept covered with dry, superfine flour, some say Buckwheat flour acts most favorably. The diet should be very spare. Eat as little as possible, until the disease begins to subside.

A very important part of the treatment of this affection is to keep the patient in a room that is comfortably warm, say at a temperature of from 65 to 75°, and keep the temperature *uniformly the same*, as nearly as possible, night and day. Do not, by any means, expose him suddenly to cold air, or a cold breeze, as on going into a cold room, going out into cold air, or undressing or dressing in a cold room. Uniformly warm temperature is of great importance.

Burns and Scalds.

No matter what the nature and extent of the burn may be, the very best of all medicines of which I have any knowledge, is *Soap*. If the parts affected, are immediately immersed or enveloped in Soft Soap, the pain will be greatly lessened, and the inflam [Pg 65] mation that would otherwise follow, will be essentially modified, if not entirely prevented. It acts like magic; no one who has never tried it can have any idea of its potency for the relief of pain, together with the prevention of bad consequences following severe burning. Under the influence of the *Soap* applications, burns and scalds will often be rendered comparatively insignificant injuries. Instead of endangering the life of the sufferer from the excessive pain, or the ulceration, or gangrene and sloughing that would follow if the pain in the first instance does not destroy life, the pain ceases, or becomes bearable in a short time, and either little or no suppuration or sloughing takes place, or the sore assumes the appearance of healthy suppuration, and heals kindly—avoiding those unsightly deformities that so commonly follow severe burning. If practicable, the soap, as before suggested, should be applied immediately after the burn, the sooner the better. The part may be put into soft soap, or cloths saturated with it can be wrapped around or covered over the affected surface, to any desirable [Pg 66] extent. The parts should not be exposed to the air for a single moment, when possible to prevent it. During the first two or three days, dressings need not be removed, unless they cause irritation after the first severe pain has subsided. They should be kept all of the time moist, and as far as practicable, in a condition to be impervious to the air.

When it is necessary to remove them, let the affected surface be immersed in strong soap suds, at a temperature of about 75 or 80°, and the dressing removed while it is under water, and others applied while in the same situation. In ordinary cases, however, even of extensive burns, after the fever consequent upon it has subsided, and the part is tolerably free from pain and smarting, the dressings may be removed in the air, but others should be in readiness and applied as speedily as possible. The soap dressings are to be continued from the beginning until the inflammation has subsided and the sore has lost all symptoms that distinguish it from an ordinary healthy suppurating sore. [Pg 67]

After the first few days, or in case of a slight burn at the beginning, an excellent mode of applying the soap, is to make a strong thick "*Lather*" with soft water and good soap, such as Castile, or any other good hard soap, as a barber would for shaving, and apply that to the affected part with a soft shaving brush; apply it as carefully as possible, so as to cover every part of the surface, and go over it several times, letting the former coat dry a little before applying another, forming a thick crust impervious to the air. In small burns, and even in pretty extensive and severe ones, this is the best mode of application, and the only one necessary.

In many cases of very severe and dangerous burns, under the influence of this application, the inflammation subsides, and after a week or more, the crust of lather comes off, exposing the surface smooth and well. Although it is important to apply the *soap* early, and the case does much better if that has been done, still I have found it the best remedy even as late as the second or third day. In such a case, the *lather* application is the best. [Pg 68]

For the fever and general nervous disturbance, *Aconite* and *Bell.* should be given alternately, as often as every half hour, and the *Aconite* should be given in appreciable doses; it acts powerfully as an anodyne. The soap treatment, or at least, the mode of applying it was first suggested to me by Dr. J. Tifft, of Norwalk, Ohio, some six or seven years ago, since which time I have had opportunities of testing its virtues in all forms of burns and scalds, some of which were of the severest and most dangerous character, and I am quite sure in several cases, no other remedy or process known to the medical profession, could have relieved and restored as this did.

The application of finely pulverized common salt, triturated with an equal part of superfine flour, acts very beneficially on burns. It seems to have the specific effect to "extract the heat," literally putting out the fire. It is particularly useful for deep burns where the surface is abraded. Some may suppose this would be severe and cause too much pain when applied to a raw surface, but so far from that being the case, [Pg 69] it is a most soothing application. It often so changes the condition of even the severest burns, in a short time, as to render them of no more importance and no more dangerous than ordinary abrasions to the same extent, by causes unconnected with heat. *Urtica urens* is directed for burns, and is useful, but the *Urtica dioica* is better. For

Chilblains,

That follow freezing or chilling the feet, causing most distressing uneasiness and itching of the feet and toes, take these remedies, *Rhus* and *Apis*, the former at night and the latter in the morning. In bad cases, they should be used once in six hours. Applications of *Oil of Arnica* to the affected parts at night, warming them before a fire, will serve greatly to palliate the sufferings, and frequently effect a perfect cure. The *Urtica Dioica* will relieve recent cases, immediately, and is one of the best remedies for the chronic affection. It should be taken at the 2d dilution, and the tincture applied to the affected part every night. [Pg 70]

Hoarseness.

This arises generally, from inflammation of the mucous membrane of the *Larynx*, in ordinary cases but slight. It is a frequent accompaniment of Bronchitis.

The remedies most useful, and those which will, in almost all ordinary cases, remove this affection at once, are *Arum tri.* and *Copaiva*, to be taken a dose every three hours in alternation.

If there is present a dry hacking cough, it will be well to take *Bell.* in the interval between the other medicines, for a day, or until the cough is relieved, or changed to a moist condition.

Inflammation of the Brain.

Brain Fever.

Though this affection is not strictly what is called "brain fever," it is attended with more or less general fever, while in what is called "Brain fever," there is great irritation of the brain, requiring in many respects similar treatment. As the treatment proper for inflammation of the brain, with some slight modifications in relation to the exist [Pg 71] ing fever, will be applicable to both, I shall treat of them under one head.

Some of the principal symptoms are delirium and drowsiness, fullness of the blood vessels of the head, beating of the temporal arteries, redness and fullness of the face, the pupils dilated, (though in the very early stage they may be contracted.) If the membranes of the brain be the seat of the disease, the pain is more intense, and frequently the limbs are in a palsied state. The patient sometimes vomits immoderately, and the pulse is slow and irregular, but full. The breathing becomes stertorous. The fever is very considerable, and the head hot.

TREATMENT.

Aconite, *Belladonna* and *Bryonia* should be given in rotation, one dose every hour in a violent case, lengthening the intervals as the symptoms abate. Applying *hot cloths* to the head, removing them occasionally to let the water evaporate, will greatly palliate and will not in the least, interrupt the action of the medicines. Never apply cold to the head of any person, when hot or inflamed, [Pg 72] much less to that of a child. Children are often killed by the application of ice to the head, producing congestion and paralysis of the brain. Hot applications are Homœopathic to the state then existing, and always beneficial. The feet may also be placed in hot water, but children should never be put into a hot or warm bath when sick, so as to cover more than the lower extremities.

Convulsions of Children—Fits.

These generally occur, either from the irritation of worms, or as precursors of ague, or they may arise from diarrhœal irritation, affecting the brain. They sometimes occur in hooping cough.

If convulsions occur from worms, the child appearing to be choked, give at once some salt and water, and as soon as the first paroxysm is over, give a dose of *Bell.*, and after an hour a dose of *Santonine*. If they come on at the commencement of an ague chill, give *Aconite* and *Bell.* every half hour for three or four doses alternately, then leave off the *Bell.* and give *Baptisia*. If diarrhœa is the cause, give *Bell.* and *Cham* [Pg 73] *omilla*. If from hooping cough, *Bell.* alone should be used.

Measles.

This is a contagious disease, and always begins with symptoms like a cold, with high fever, and a severe dry cough, thirst and restlessness. *Pulsatilla* is the proper medicine to palliate and regulate the symptoms. If the fever is high, *Aconite* should be used every two hours alternately with *Puls.* Should the eruption subside suddenly, give *Bryonia* with *Pulsatilla* until it reappears.

Let the child drink freely of cold water, and avoid stimulants of every kind. If the eruption is tardy in its appearance, a hot bath may be administered, being careful to have the room quite warm, and to rub the patient dry, very suddenly after the bath. Frictions by the healthy hand over the surface, will do much towards bringing out measles. After the eruption is out, quiet, freedom from sudden exposure to cold, cold water and light diet is all that is necessary. In some of the most obstinate cases, where [Pg 74] the eruptions failed to appear in the proper time, as well as where they had receded too soon, I have been able to bring them out in a short time with an infusion of Sassafras root, sweetened and taken quite warm, in doses of half an ounce in fifteen to thirty minutes. It is a remedy for measles well worth attention.

Mumps.

This is a contagious disease, consisting in an inflammation of the Parotid gland. There is, at first, a sense of stiffness and soreness on moving the jaw, soon after the gland begins to swell, and continues to be sore and painful, with more or less headache, and general fever for from six to eight days. It is not ordinarily a dangerous disease, unless translated to some other part. It may remove from the original seat to the brain, the testicles, or in females to the breasts.

TREATMENT.

Mercurius should be given three times a day during the attack. If the brain becomes affected, use *Bell.* and *Apis mel.* in [Pg 75] alternation. Should it recede to the testicles, or to the female breasts, *Apis mel.* is *the* remedy. *Mercurius* may be used in connection with the *Apis* as soon as the violent symptoms have subsided, in order to prevent permanent glandular swellings.

Stings of Insects.

The effect produced by the sting of Bees, Wasps, and Hornets of all kinds, is so nearly, if not quite identical, that I shall make no distinction between them. There are very few, if any persons, who do not know the symptoms, at least the local effects of the Bee sting. Pungent, stinging, aching pain, redness and swelling of the part. The wound has at first, and for some time, a white spot or point where the sting entered, surrounded by an areola of bright scarlet, growing fainter and paler as it recedes. The swelling is not pointed, but a rounded elevation, with a feeling of hardness. If upon the face, it not unfrequently causes the whole face to swell so as to nearly if not entirely close the eyes. In some instances, the brain becomes affected and death ensues. [Pg 76]

TREATMENT.

I have for many years, used but *one remedy*, and that has in all cases, and under all circumstances, when applied at any stage of the affection, produced prompt and perfect relief; therefore I shall recommend no other. It is the common garden *Onion*, (*Allium cepa*) applied to the spot where the sting entered. I cut the fresh Onion and apply the raw surface to the spot, changing it for a fresh piece every ten to fifteen minutes, until the pain and swelling, and all disagreeable symptoms disappear. If it is applied immediately after the stinging, the first application will afford perfect relief in a few minutes, and no further effect from it will be experienced. Applied later, it must be continued longer, and this may be done one or two days after the stinging, with just as much certainty of removing whatever symptoms may still exist.

I treated one case when three days had elapsed, the patient (a young lady) was delirious and speechless, the whole face was so swollen as to entirely disfigure her features, raising the cheeks to a level with the [Pg 77] nose, and closing the eyes. Her life was almost despaired of. The surface of a freshly cut onion was applied to the point where the sting entered, and changed about once an hour for a fresh piece. In a few hours consciousness returned, and a rapid recovery followed. All the swelling and disagreeable symptoms were gone in three days.

Ledum is highly recommended by some Physicians, and is doubtless of some value, but it is not to be compared with the *Allium*.

The most potent and certain remedy for the poison caused by the

Bite of the Rattlesnake

is *Alcohol*, in the ordinary form, or in common Whisky, Brandy, Rum or Gin. Let the patient drink it freely, a gill or more at a time, once in fifteen to twenty minutes, until some symptoms of intoxication are experienced, then cease using it. The cure will be complete as soon as enough has been taken to produce even slight symptoms of intoxication. It is remarkable how much [Pg 78] alcohol a patient suffering from the poison of the Rattlesnake will bear.

An intelligent medical friend of mine in Kanawha County, Virginia, gave a little girl of ten years, who had been bitten by a Rattlesnake, over three quarts of good strong Whisky, in less than a day, when but slight symptoms of intoxication were produced, and that seemed to arise entirely from the last drink. She recovered from the intoxication in a few hours, and suffered no more from the poison of the serpent.

Instances of cures with whisky are numerous, and I have never heard of a failure, when it was used as here directed. I presume it will do the same for the poison of other serpents.

Headache.

This symptom or affection, (if it can be classed as a disease) may depend upon so many causes, and be so very different in its effects, degrees of intensity, and the kind of pain or sensation attending it, that one will find it very difficult to mark out any definite treatment. I shall, therefore, only point [Pg 79] out some of the more frequent cases, and the indications for certain remedies.

What is called "*sick headache*," or "nervous headache," begins by a sense of blindness or blur, before the eyes, of green or purple colors, dazzling or swimming in the head, without, for some time at first, any positive aching or pain. In the course of an hour, a longer or shorter time, the dimness of vision goes off, and the head begins to ache. This may or may not be accompanied with nausea and vomiting. Some persons are always more or less sick at the stomach, when these "nervous headaches" come on, others are not thus affected.

TREATMENT.

If taken as soon as the first blur before the eyes is noticed, or before any pain is felt in the head, *Nux Vomica* will, in nearly all cases, arrest the disease at once. It may be necessary to take two or three doses at intervals of an hour. Later in the case, though *Nux* may palliate, it will not cure.

If headache with sickness comes on, *Macrotin* and *Podoph.* should be given in alterna [Pg 80] tion, every half hour, if the symptoms are very severe, and the nausea great; but in a mild case, give it once an hour, lengthening the interval as the symptoms abate.

If the feet are cold, as is often the case, putting them into hot water will palliate the symptoms, and not interfere with the medicines.

If the head feels hot, apply *hot* water to it. Never apply cold to the head, when there are any symptoms of congestion, as of fullness of the blood vessels. For

Common Headache,

If the face is red, and the arteries of the neck and temples throb violently, give *Bell*. If there is paleness and faintness, *Pulsatilla* is the remedy, especially if the forehead is principally affected. If the pain is mostly in the back of the head, *Nux* is to be used; if in the front, and is sharp, affecting the eyes, *Aconite*; if at the angles of the forehead, with a sense of pinching, *Arnica*; if a sense of fullness and pressing outwards, or with an enlarged feeling, *Macrotin*; if intermitting or remitting, *Mercurius*; if there is ringing [Pg 81] in the ears, *China*. Headache from fright should have *Aconite*.

For that kind of *headache* that often occurs during the prevalence of fevers, and is not unfrequently a premonitory symptom of an attack of fever, I have found *Baptisia* and *Podophyllin* to be specifics. I give them alternately, every two hours a dose, until the headache ceases. It often subsides in a few minutes after the first dose of either, though I have sometimes failed with one alone and succeeded in the same cases afterwards with both in alternation. *I have no doubt* but that they act in many cases, as *Prophylactics*, entirely warding off and preventing fevers, or at least arresting them at the premonitory stage. *Podophyllin* is a most valuable remedy for headache.

Nose Bleed—Epistaxis.

If it arises from fullness of the vessels of the head, with throbbing of the temples, redness of the face and eyes, *Belladonna* is the remedy. If fever is present, *Aconite* must be alternated with *Bell.*

In females or children who have habitual [Pg 82] nose-bleed, *Pulsatilla* and *Podophyllin* are to be used alternately, night and morning. During the paroxysm of bleeding, *Arnica* should be used, one dose repeated in a half hour if it continues.

If it is produced by over-exertion, *Rhus* is the proper remedy. If it occurs in the *early stage* of fever, *Aconite* and *Bell.*; in the latter stage, *Rhus* and *Phos.* are to be used. *Hamamelis* will frequently arrest nose-bleed *immediately* after one or two doses.

Worms.

It is difficult to determine the presence of *worms* in children, much more in adults, yet both are affected by them occasionally. In children, there is more or less fever and restlessness, screaming out in sleep, starting, pain in the bowels, vomiting, choking, diarrhœa, picking at the nose, fetid breath, voracious and variable appetite.

TREATMENT.

Santonine is a remedy which I have used for years, and I have treated many hundreds of cases, with such unvariable success, that I feel disinclined to use or to recommend [Pg 83] any other. It brings away the worms entire, and relieves the patient of all morbid symptoms immediately, or in much less time than any other remedy of which I have any knowledge. It seems to act specifically upon the worms, causing them to leave the bowels by being evacuated with the feces, without producing any sensible impression upon the bowels, the evacuations remaining natural, if they were so, or becoming so, if deranged, and the worms coming away not quite lifeless.

I have often prescribed this remedy for children suffering under intermittent or remitting, and even typhoid fever, in the summer season, when there were not present any well defined symptoms of worms, and yet the fever would soon abate, and in due time worms appear in the fecal evacuations. It often arrests entirely intermittent fever, when worms are present, and are the probable cause of the fever.

I give either the crude salt in from one-fourth to one-half grain doses, or a trituration of one grain to four of sugar, giving in the latter case, from one to two grains of the tritu [Pg 84] ration. Give one dose at bed-time, or in an urgent case at any other time, but never repeat the dose under thirty-six hours, and in an ordinary case, under forty-eight hours.

This is *the* medicine *par excellence* for worms. It may be repeated once a week, when there is a tendency in the patient to the development of worm symptoms, or, in other words, the breeding of worms. The idea held out by some that it is hurtful, or unimportant to remove the worms, in itself considered, is simply *nonsense*, and *worse*, for children are sometimes sacrificed to this idea.

Earache—Otalgia.

This may arise from various causes, but a common one is sudden cold. If it arises from cold, and there is general fever, or if the ear is red, or the side of the head and ear hot, *Bell.* and *Baptisia* should be given in alternation, every hour, or in a violent case, more frequently. These remedies will soon relieve such cases. Cloths wrung out of hot water should be laid over the ear, or the side of the head steamed, or it may be laid into water quite warm, with good effect.

Where the disease is a chronic affection, and the patient is subject to frequent attacks of pain in the ear, especially on a change of the weather, from dry to moist, *Mercurius* is the proper remedy, especially if it is worse at night, when warm in bed.

If it arises from a shock or blow, *Arn.* is to be used. In scrofulous persons, whether there is ulceration or not, *Phosphorus* and *Pulsatilla* are the remedies.

Children and even adults, not unfrequently suffer from earache, without any known cause sufficient to account for it. On examination into the ear you will often find either the cavity filled or nearly so, with a hard black substance, (the inspissated "earwax") almost as hard as horn, or else the ear will be quite empty, and the sides of the cavity *dry* and red, though perhaps not properly in a state of inflammation.

The natural condition of the cavity as it can be seen by straining the ear outwards and backwards a little in a strong sun light, is moist, the surface covered slightly with a yellowish, greasy, soft substance (the cerumen) "earwax." When this is wanting or in excess, or its character changed, it is evidence of disease, and pain is likely to occur. The

TREATMENT

for this condition is to remove the accumulation when that exists, as the first step. But this must be first softened by pouring some warm oil, pure olive oil, or good pure sperm oil, into the ear, and repeat it two or three times a day for several days, until it is so far softened as to be easily removed with the probe end of common small tweezers, having a spoon-bowl point.

When there is dryness, moisten the surface with oil. In either case, it is best, for a while, to protect the delicate surface from the air, by putting oiled wool into the external ear.

If the ear was filled, give *Mercurius* once a day until there appears a natural secretion. If dry, use *Belladonna*.

Toothache.

It is difficult to determine the cause of toothache, and more difficult to select the remedy. It often depends upon decay of [Pg 87] the tooth, and exposure of the nerve to air, and contact with food or drinks, or even saliva, which irritate and produce pain.

Pulsatilla will as often relieve such cases as any other remedy, yet if it has been aggravated by a recent cold, *Bell.* and *Nux V.* may be better. If the nerve is not exposed, and there is a disposition to a return of the pain on exposure to cold air, or a change of weather, the pain being of a *rheumatic* character, give *Rhus* and *Macrotin* in alternation. These will relieve many cases. For decayed teeth, the pain being dull aching, with soreness, use *Chamomilla*. The body of the tooth, that is the dentine, sometimes becomes very sensitive when there is no decay or cavity, the pain being experienced when some hard substance hits, or the air or water, either cold or hot, comes in contact with the tooth. The temporary pain will generally yield to *Arnica*, and in most instances, the daily use of *Arnica* at the first decimal dilution, applied to the surface, and upon the jaws, will effect a cure.

The *chloride of Zinc* applied to the surface of such teeth for a few moments will [Pg 88] destroy the sensitiveness of the dentine.

Teeth that are ulcerated at the roots, or have ulcerated gums around them, the teeth being decayed, should be extracted at once, for, besides the pain and inconvenience they cause, they are a *very prolific* source of *disturbance* to the digestive organs, from the positive poison generated by the decaying process.

If people will use soft brushes upon the teeth with soap and water, followed by rinsing with simple water only, after each meal, brushing both inside and out and crossways, so as to clean between them, they will be saved much pain and decay, and disease of other parts, arising from foul and diseased teeth.

Teething of Children.

Affections arising from teething of children, are often of a serious character. The most prominent of which is *Diarrhœa*. *Fever* frequently accompanies the diarrhœa, and *convulsions* occasionally occur. *Aconite* and *Chamomilla* should be used in alternation, every one or two hours, according to [Pg 89] the violence of the fever, and if convulsions occur, or are threatened, as will be known by twitching, starting, and screaming, use *Nux* and *Bell*. These may be given in rotation with the others, following the remedies, one after the other, every hour. I have relieved the most alarming cases in a day by this method of procedure, that had not yielded to either of the single remedies for several days, given as directed in the books; the patient growing worse continually. If the gums over the teeth look white and the teeth, (one or more,) are near the surface, the gums should, by all means, be cut. Press the point of a lancet or penknife down upon the top of the gum, until the tooth is plainly felt, and be sure to make the cut as wide as the tooth. Rub the gums with *Arnicated water* once or twice a day. *Pulsatilla* should be given at night and *Chamomilla* in the morning, during the whole summer while the child is teething, as a prophylactic against the fever and diarrhœa that is likely to occur. It will generally save all trouble. [Pg 90]

If the diarrhœa is profuse, watery and light colored or brown, give *Phos. acid* and *Veratrum* alternately, as often as the discharges occur. For the restlessness of infants at night, *Coffea* is the specific.

Apthæ—Thrush.

This is a disease peculiar to nursing children. The mouth becomes sore, and the tongue, lips, and fauces are covered with a white crust, looking like milk curds, which, when removed, leaves the surface red, inflamed and very tender. It sooner or later, extends to the stomach and bowels, producing severe and dangerous diarrhœa.

TREATMENT.

Of all the medicines known to our Materia Medica, none, according to my experience, will in the least, compare with the *Eupatorium aromaticum*. It is almost, if not quite certain to relieve speedily in all cases. I say this, not only from my own experience and observation, but from the testimony of several other Homœopathic Physicians, who have, within the last year, used it. [Pg 91]

It should be given at the first or second dilution, once in four or six hours, and three or four drops of the tincture put into a teaspoonful of water, and the mouth occasionally washed with the mixture.

In summer, where agues prevail, and the child is feverish and restless, *China* will aid in the cure, to be given once in six hours between the doses of the *Eupatorium*. If the diarrhœa is obstinate, the discharges colored, and the child is sick at the stomach, give *Podophyllin* with the other remedies.

Inflammation of the Eyes—Ophthalmia.

For common Ophthalmia, in the early stages, while there is more or less fever and headache, with flushed face, bloodshot eyes and throbbing of the temporal arteries, *Bell.* and *Aconite* should be used alternately every two hours, and a wash made with ten drops of tincture of Aconite to one gill of pure water, applied to the eyes as hot as the patient can bear. This application should be repeated every two hours, in a violent case, until the eyes are easy, and then about twice a day until all inflammation and red [Pg 92] ness pass off. This will relieve a large proportion of cases in from one to four days.

If, however, the case continues obstinate for a longer time, or has been of a week or more standing before the treatment is commenced, in the place of Bell., or after using it one or two days, use *Hydrastus* with the *Aconite*, giving them alternately at intervals of two to six hours, according to the stage of the case—more frequently as the symptoms are more urgent, using washes prepared of each separately, as directed for Aconite, except that the Hydrastus wash may be twice as strong; and apply each about half as often as the same medicine is taken internally. The wash should, in all cases of acute inflammation of the eyes, be as hot as it can be borne. Let it be put into the eyes so as to come directly in contact with the inflamed surface.

Simple hot water applied to inflamed eyes for hours together, allowing short intervals between the applications, will often cure most painful cases.

Never apply cold to inflamed eyes. It always aggravates. When the inflammation [Pg 93] is in a scrofulous person, especially in infants, it assumes a purulent character, and may leave the cornea in clouded (nebulous) condition, and the sight more or less obliterated. For this condition use *Conium* first, and apply it *in tinct.*, half water, to the eyes every four hours.

Wounds and Bruises.

On this subject, I must necessarily be very brief. When a wound is inflicted, the first and most important thing to be done is to *arrest the flow of blood*. Every one should know how to do this. The bleeding is to be stopped, and the wounded vessels to be secured, so that no further flow can take place.

First, then, to stop the bleeding, *pressure* is to be made upon the artery leading to the wound. If the wound is in the leg or foot, pressure is to be made, either on the vessel above and near the wound, or, where that cannot be easily found and compressed, make firm pressure with the thumb or some hard substance, in the groin, about two and a half inches at one side of the center of the pelvis, (wounded side) just below the lower [Pg 94] margin of the belly, towards the inner side of the thigh, where the great artery (Femoral artery) can be felt pulsating. By pressing firmly upon this artery, the blood is arrested in its flow into the limb, and of course the bleeding from the wound soon ceases. If the wound is in the arm or hand, *pressure* is to be made, either just above the wound, or on the inside of the arm, about one-third of the way from the shoulder to the elbow, where the artery (Brachial) can be felt. To secure the parts from further bleeding, the wounded artery must be taken up and tied. Let it be seized by forceps, or the point of a needle may be thrust into it, and the vessel stretched out a little, a thread put round it and tied; cut off one end of the tie, and let the other hang out of the wound, until it comes out by the vessel sloughing off. Bring the lips of the wound together, and if it is large, put in stitches enough to hold them, and put on an adhesive plaster, compress of cloths, and bandages to keep it from straining the stitches, and protect it from the air. The *Arnica* plaster, made by John Hall, of Cleveland, is the best adhesive plaster of [Pg 95] which I have any knowledge. Give the patient *Aconite* once in two hours, for a day after the accident.

Slight Cuts about the joints, especially the knee, are dangerous, from their liability to affect the ligaments, inflame, and produce *Lockjaw*. Therefore, such wounds, ever so slight, are of great importance. They should be at once closed up, whether they bleed or not, and covered with an adhesive plaster, (Arnica plaster is the best) a bandage, and the knee should not be bent, even when walking or sitting, until the wound is healed. It is best to apply a splint from the hip to the heel, and bandage the limb to it, so as to prevent bending of the joint.

Bruises are to be treated with *Arnica*, applied to the part affected, by putting twenty drops of the tincture into a gill of water, if the skin is *not* ruptured, or three drops into the same if it is, and bathing freely. The *Arnica* is to be taken internally at a higher dilution. Keep the parts covered with cloths and wet in *Arnica* water. [Pg 96]

If a blow is received upon the head, by a fall, or in any other way, producing a "stunning" effect, (concussion of the brain) so that the patient appears lifeless for a time, and delirious when he begins to come to, there is great danger of inflammation of the brain, and death from the re-action, or in some cases, the shock is so great that the patient will never revive unless he has the proper aid.

Arnica is the great remedy to bring on reaction, arouse the patient, and prevent *dangerous* inflammation or congestion of the brain.

When a patient is "stunned" by a blow or fall, he should be conveyed soon as possible, to some *quiet* place, and as little noise as practicable made about him, and the room kept darkened. *Arnica* 3d should be given immediately, and the nostrils wet with strongly arnicated water.

If fever arise after he comes to, *Aconite* should be given with *Arnica*, and if the head aches, or becomes hot, *Bell.* is to be used. This will prevent or arrest all symptoms of inflammation. [Pg 97]

Torn and Mangled wounds should not be handled much. If they bleed, the blood must be stopped as in any other case. If they are dirty, warm water may be gently applied to cleanse them. The wound should be covered with some soft cloths, and kept constantly wet in Arnicated water of the strength of four drops of the *tincture* to a pint of water.

Piles — Hemorrhoids.

One important matter in all cases of habitual piles, is, to keep the bowels regular. Much can be done for this purpose by diet and regimen. On rising from bed in the morning drink freely, from a gill to half a pint of cold water, at least half an hour before breakfast; use such diet as is easily digested, and drink no alcoholic beverages. To relieve the bowels when costive, take a dose of *Nux Vomica* at night, and *Podophyllin* in the morning. This may be repeated from day to day until the proper effect is produced.

To relieve from a severe attack of Piles, use *Bell.* and *Podophyllin* in alternation [Pg 98] every four hours, and apply to the tumors when inflamed, cloths wrung out of hot water, or sit in hot water for a time.

A poultice made of fine-cut *Tobacco* wet in hot water and crowded firmly up against the pile-tumors, secured by a T bandage, will relieve the most desperate cases for the time, and is attended with no danger or disagreeable symptoms except in rare cases, when it produces sickness at the stomach, which soon subsides on the poultice being removed. *Oil of Arnica* is an excellent application for inflamed Piles.

A most important point in the management of Piles, and one often neglected, is to replace the prolapsed tumors. The tumors will be protruded from within the anus by the act of evacuating, and if left in that condition, will be pressed upon by the external parts, chafed and inflamed. In all such cases, the patient should take particular pains to return the tumors into the rectum; and to aid in that process a little oil may be applied when they will be easily pushed back, and the sphincter of the bowel will close below [Pg 99] them, preventing any chafing, and the consequent inflammation.

For *Bleeding Piles, Ipecac* and *Bell.* are very efficient remedies. They may be alternated every half hour, or oftener if the bleeding is severe, or at longer intervals when it is only slight.

Hamamelis V., (Witch Hazel,) will in nearly all cases arrest the bleeding at once. It should be applied to the parts and taken internally at the same time. Drop doses to be put on the tongue once in fifteen or twenty minutes.

An infusion of the *Hamamelis* may be taken internally in doses of half a teaspoonful, and the same injected into the bowel with excellent effect.

The most effectual way, and the best for obtaining permanent relief from Piles when the tumors have become hard, and remain all the time so as to pass out of the anus at every evacuation, being constantly more or less tender and painful, and often becoming inflamed, is to have them taken off. But never let that be done with a knife. The bleeding would, in such a case, be very [Pg 100] excessive, and most likely fatal. The history of knife operations for the excision of Pile tumors is written in blood, and the tombstone stands as a monument of condemnation of the practice. No trustworthy surgeon will at this day attempt it.

But however dangerous may be the knife operation, there is no danger at all to be apprehended from removing the tumors by a *ligature*. To accomplish this, take a soft cork about three-fourths of an inch in diameter, and one inch long—make a hole through the center from end to end, about one-eighth of an inch in diameter—cut crucial grooves in the top of the cork about an eighth of an inch deep, bevel down the lower end nearly to an edge, make a cord of saddler's silk, three fold twisted together and waxed, about eight or ten inches long, double this in the middle and pass the loop down through the cork out at the sharp end, the two loose ends of the string being out at the grooved end. Make a strong hickory stick about three-sixteenths of an inch in diameter, and just long enough to pass across the square end of the cork. Now have the [Pg 101] patient protrude the Pile tumors as far out as possible, being placed on his knees with the head bent to the floor, pressing out firmly as if to evacuate the bowels. Let the tumors be dried as much as possible by gently pressing a soft, dry cloth to them; then let the loop of the string projecting from the flattened end of the cork, be pushed on over the largest tumor, and held down at its base, while an assistant places the stick in one of the grooves, ties the two ends of the cord firmly down over the stick, or *toggle*, by a square bow knot; then turn the stick round once, twice, or more, until the pressure upon the tumor is sufficient to strangulate it perfectly, and prevent the string from slipping off. Care should be taken to keep the cord down to the base of the tumor while it is being tied and tightened, as in many cases the base is much the larger part of the tumor, and the cord tends to slip up. After the ligature is applied and tightened, apply arnicated water to the parts, and a large, warm poultice of superfine slippery elm bark, wet so as not to be too soft and slippery, on the face of which Arnica may be put. Keep [Pg 102] it on with a T bandage. The patient must be put to bed and kept quiet until the ligature and tumor come off, which will be in about six or seven days, sometimes sooner. Once a day the "toggle" must be turned part, or the whole of a circle or more, to tighten the cord as the patient can bear. This will be very painful from beginning to end of the ligating, but any, even the most sensitive, patient can bear it. The patient must have quite warm hip baths two, three, or more, times a day, or as often as the pain is severe, the poultice being replaced after each bath, and kept constantly on.

If there are several tumors protruding, apply ligatures to two of the largest, when these are removed, the others will disappear.

Injections of mucillage of slippery elm should be carefully used to move the bowels daily, or at least once in two days. Let the diet be of corn or oat meal mush, or rice. As the tumor gradually sloughs off, the surface heals, so that, though the base where the ligature was applied, may have been an inch or more across it, there will not be a raw surface of over an eighth of an inch in diam [Pg 103] eter, to which *Calendula Cerate* should be applied. The patient must keep quiet for a few days longer. Though this is a painful operation, it is not in the slightest degree dangerous. I have effected complete and permanent cures by this mode in numerous instances.

Sea-Sickness.

Nux Vomica should be used once in about four hours, for twelve hours before sailing, as a preventive to sea-sickness.

If, however, symptoms, such as dizziness or blur before the eyes, and headache, begin to come on, a dose of *Nux* should be taken, followed in an hour with *Pulsatilla*.

If the nausea comes on, *Ipecac* and *Arsenicum* should be taken alternately between the paroxysms of vomiting, should that symptom appear.

If practicable, the patient should lay still upon the back until the sickness passes off. I have removed sea-sickness immediately in several instances with *Pulsatilla* alone, and the last time I had an opportunity to prescribe for this affection I gave *Podophyllin*. It removed all the symptoms in a few [Pg 104] minutes. That is the only time I ever tried it, but from the provings I am satisfied it is one of the best remedies.

Asiatic Cholera.

I was practicing in Cincinnati during the prevalence of Cholera in the years 1849, and 1850, and in Northern Ohio in 1854, and had abundant opportunity to observe and treat it. The disease generally begins with a diarrhœa, which may continue for several days, or only a few hours before other symptoms set in, such as vomiting, then cramping in the stomach and muscles of the legs, arms, hands and feet, followed by cold sweats, great prostration, restlessness, excessive and burning thirst, drinks being immediately rejected. These symptoms continue, the patient sinking rapidly into *collapse*, when the skin looks blue and shriveled, the eyes sunken, the surface covered with a cold, clammy sweat, the extremities, nose, ears, tongue and breath cold, the voice hollow and unnatural. This condition continues from two to eight or ten hours, the patient regularly failing, sometimes becoming delirious before he dies. [Pg 105]

In some cases the vomiting and diarrhœa set in simultaneously, and the other symptoms follow, as above described, in rapid succession. In others the cramping may be the first symptom, the others following it.

In a large proportion of cases, the disease takes the course first described above, the diarrhœa, called the *premonitory symptoms*, or sometimes *cholerine*, coming on several hours, if not a day or more, before any other symptoms.

The diarrhœa is not usually painful, hence the patient may not be alarmed so as to attend to it until the more dangerous symptoms appear. It begins in some cases with pain and some griping, the discharges rather consistent, having a bilious appearance, so that the patient supposes it to be an ordinary bilious diarrhœa, which is not dangerous, his fears being thus quieted. But however the diarrhœa begins, it becomes sooner or later, copious, watery, and light colored, (rice water) painless but rapidly prostrating.

TREATMENT.

In the early stages of the diarrhœa, *Veratrum*, taken about twice as often as the evac [Pg 106] uations occur, will frequently arrest it in a few hours, especially if the patient lies down and keeps quiet. But if not, and it increases in frequency, or becomes more copious, or any sickness is felt at the stomach, the patient should, at once, be laid upon a bed and *strong tincture of Camphor* should be given in drop doses, once in five minutes, for one hour or more, and as the symptoms abate, once in ten, fifteen or twenty minutes, for six or eight hours.

A teaspoonful of the *Camphor tincture* may be put into a tumbler of cold water, ice water if at hand, and the water agitated until it becomes clear, giving a teaspoonful of this camphorated *cold* water as a dose, stirring the water each time. I think this is better than to give the pure tincture. After the patient becomes quiet and easy, *Veratrum* should be given in alternation with Camphor, a dose in four to six hours for several days, or oftener if he feels any symptoms like a threatened return of the disease. These two medicines serve as *prophylactics* (preventives) of Cholera. [Pg 107]

If, however, the disease continues in spite of the Camphor and Veratrum, in the first instance, or later, (as the Camphor may be given in many cases with success in the advance stage,) you must resort to other remedies.

If vomiting comes on with burning in the stomach give *Ipecac* and *Arsenicum* in alternation as often as the vomiting occurs, and if the diarrhœa continues give *Veratrum* between the doses of the other two, in a violent case, as often as every ten to fifteen minutes, and at longer intervals when the disease is slow in its progress. If the vomiting and diarrhœa, or either, occur with a kind of explosion, the vomiting ceasing suddenly for the time, after the first *gush*, or the discharges from the bowels are involuntary, *Secale* is the specific remedy.

For the cramping, *Cuprum* and *Veratrum* are the remedies to be given alternately.

If, however, the *cramping* comes on as the first symptom, which is sometimes the case, the patient being suddenly seized with it before any other alarming symptoms occur, *Camphor* is *the great remedy*, and in this case [Pg 108] it may be given in doses of double or treble the quantity before directed.

If he sinks into the *collapse* and lies quiet, indifferent to everything, the pulse sinking, or he is pulseless, *Carbo Veg.* will sometimes arouse and restore him, hopeless as the case appears. It should be given once in half an hour until the pulse begins to rise. If, however, instead of being quiet he is restless and thirsty, give *Arsenicum* in alternation with *Carbo Veg.*, repeating the dose as above directed. In some cases, after all the active symptoms cease, the patient will become quiet and drop to sleep, and instead of the pulse rising, as it will if he is recovering, it sinks, or does not appear if he has been pulseless, and the breathing becomes irregular and feeble—he is sinking. If aroused, he sinks back into the stupor in a few moments as before. *Laurocerasus* is a specific for this condition. It should be given once an hour until he is aroused.

If, however, besides the stupor, the head is hot, the face red, the breathing oppressed, the pulse slow and sluggish, *Opium* is to be [Pg 109] used, and may be given in alternation with *Laurocerasus*.

For the irritation of the brain, and furious delirium that sometimes sets in after the cessation of cholera symptoms, *Secale* and *Belladonna* in alternation will prove specific.

Let the patient have warm or cold drink as he prefers, and let his covering be light or plentiful as is most agreeable. As soon as he gets easy, and the vomiting and purging cease, and his pulse begins to return, keep him quiet as possible, let the room be darkened and everything still, so that he may go to sleep, which he is inclined to do, this being the surest restorer. I am quite sure I have known several patients carried off by a return of the disease, after it had been effectually arrested, in consequence of sleep being prevented by the rejoicing officiousness and congratulations of friends, disturbing and preventing that early and quiet slumber which nature so much needs, and must have, or hopelessly sink. The diet for two or three days after recovery, should be a little oat meal gruel or rice. [Pg 110]

Small Pox—Variola.

This disease begins with pain in the head and back, chilly sensations, followed by a high fever, so similar in all respects to a severe attack of Bilious or "winter" fever, that it is difficult or impossible to distinguish it with certainty, as Small Pox. The fact of the prevalence of the disease at the time, and the exposure of the patient, may lead the Physician and friends to suspect Small Pox. There is one very striking symptom of Small Pox, however, that exists from the beginning, which, though it may be present in fever simply, is not uniformly so. This is a severe and constant aching *pain in the small of the back*. The headache is also constant.

The Small Pox is of two varieties or degrees, *distinct* and *confluent*. The *distinct* is when the pustules are separated from each other, each one a distinct elevation, with more or less space between them not affected by the eruption.

The *confluent* is where the pustules spread out from their sides and run together, covering the whole surface as one sore. [Pg 111]

It may be distinct on some parts, as on the body, and confluent on others, as the arms, face, and parts most exposed to the air.

In the *Distinct* variety the fever continues without abatement until the eruption appears, when it entirely subsides, and that quite suddenly. The eruption comes out about the third day of the attack, sometimes not discoverable until the end of the third or beginning of the fourth day. The eruption is at first very slight, beginning with small red pimples on the forehead, upper part of the cheeks, neck and upper part of the breast, extending by degrees to the arms, and other parts of the body and limbs. About the end of the fourth or forepart of the fifth day, the eruption is complete.

There is a symptom, not mentioned in the books, which will often determine the disease before the occurrence of any eruption. It is the appearance of hard shot-like pimples, to be *felt under the skin* in the palms of the hands, while there is, as yet, no trace of eruption to be seen upon the surface.

On the eighth or ninth day, the eruptions become vessicular, have flattened tops, and [Pg 112] contain a limpid fluid. The parts continue to swell, the eruptions to enlarge, and become filled with purulent matter, having a dark color at the top, up to about the fourteenth or fifteenth day, when they begin to flat down, to dry up, and some of the scabs become loose. At this time, some fever arises, often quite severe, with headache and other inflammatory symptoms. If the eruption is very severe, fever will be of corresponding violence, and lighter or wanting when the eruption is mild. This fever rarely lasts more than twenty-four hours, from which time the patient rapidly recovers.

In the *Confluent* variety, all the symptoms are more violent, the fever continuing after the eruption begins. The pustules burst early, and run into each other, covering nearly or quite the whole skin; the surface swells and turns black or dark brown, the lungs are more or less irritated, producing cough, and not unfrequently the stomach is nauseated, and vomiting ensues.

If the patient survives the irritation up to the fifteenth or sixteenth day, when the *secondary fever* sets in, he is liable to be taken [Pg 113] off by an affection of the brain or lungs, during this fever. If he recovers, his whole surface, especially that part exposed to air, is deeply pitted.

TREATMENT.

As it is not often known for a certainty, in the early febrile stage, that it is the small pox, the treatment will be first adopted that would be proper for a like fever arising from other causes. But in all my observations in this disease, and they extend to several hundred cases, I have not found in a single instance, any of the ordinary fever remedies, such as *Aconite* and *Bell.*, which would be applicable for such symptoms in an ordinary case, to do any good in small pox. They are directed, however, for these symptoms by the authorities, in the febrile stage of the small pox; but I am quite sure they are not the proper remedies.

From the great similarity, the almost absolute identity of small pox *headache* and *backache*, with the same symptoms developed by the *Macrotys racem.* as well as the nausea and restlessness produced by the drug, I was led [Pg 114] several years ago to the conclusion that this, or the *Macrotin* was valuable in small pox. Not only so, but during the prevalence of small pox in Cincinnati, to an extraordinary degree in the winter of 1849-50, I treated about one hundred cases, including both sexes, and all ages, from infants a few weeks old, to very old persons, giving the *Macrotin* to all, and had the good fortune to see *all* my patients recover. Since that time I have prescribed it for every case successfully.

Having then, been entirely successful in so many cases, with this medicine, I am not inclined at this time to give any other the preference. I must admit, however, that though my patients all recovered, I was not able to greatly abridge the duration of the disease, nor to prevent the development of all the stages in their proper order, as is *claimed* by M. Teste, for his use of *Mercurius cor.* and *Causticum*. I was satisfied with so far modifying the symptoms, as to enable my patients to live through, and come *out well in the end*. I would then direct, if small pox is suspected, the patient having been exposed to contract it, or from the peculiarity of the symptoms, [Pg 115] in the early stage, or when the disease is discovered after the eruption, to give *Macrotin* at the first trituration, in one grain doses, once in two hours, while the fever, headache and backache continue, after which, during the whole course of the disease, give it three times a day. This will prevent the development of a dangerous secondary fever, as well as irritation of the lungs, stomach or bowels. In addition to this medicine I give the patients daily, from half an ounce to two ounces of *pure* (*unrancid*) *Olive oil*. This serves to prevent the development of pustules in the throat, lungs and stomach; is more or less nutritious, and keeps the bowels in a healthy condition. Wash the surface once a day in weak soap suds, following it with a bath of milk and water, and keep cloths moistened with warm milk and water, constantly upon all parts that are exposed to the air, lubricating the surface with *Olive oil* after the bath of milk and water. This keeps the surface quite comfortable.

The best diet is corn or oat meal mush and molasses, to be taken in small quantities. [Pg 116] Cold water is the proper drink, though it should not be very cold.

The room should, at all times, be well ventillated, but in cold or cool weather, sufficient fire must be kept up, to keep the room warm and dry. A temperature of about 65° is the best. Hardly any thing can be worse for a small pox patient than to be in a cold or damp room, and to breathe *cold* air. Uniform temperature is important.

If the eruption is tardy about appearing, or after it is out, a recession takes place, the Alcoholic Vapor bath will soon bring it out. (See Rheumatism p. **30**).

Occasionally the feet and limbs below the knees, will swell prodigiously, and become extremely painful, causing the principal suffering. For this, wrap the feet and legs in cloths wet in a strong solution of Epsom salts, quite warm, and cover with flannels so as to keep them warm. This will afford immediate relief, and reduce the swelling in a day or two. The finely pulverized Epsom salts, dry, sprinkled on the pustules, will very often prevent pitting. It is the safest and surest remedy of which I have any knowledge. [Pg 117]

Varioloid

is small pox modified by vaccination. It is to be treated as a mild case of small pox. The *Macrotin* has been used with apparent success as a prophylactic (preventive) to small pox, taken three times daily.

Painful Urination, Incontinence of Urine,

Involuntary Urination.

Where the discharge of urine produces smarting and burning of the urethra, *Cantharis* is the remedy. Where there seems to be an over secretion of acrid urine, producing inflammation of the neck of the bladder, known by pain in the glans penis, *Copaiva*, and *Apis mel.* are the remedies. If there appears to be a partial palsy of the neck of the bladder, the discharge taking place in sleep, *Podophyllin* is the surest remedy. I have cured some bad cases by the use of these three remedies, given in rotation three or four hours apart.

Injections of a solution of borax into the bladder, have, in several cases, been sufficient to effect a perfect cure, without any other remedy. This may be used in con [Pg 118] nection with the other remedies. For painful urination with a distressed feeling in the neck of the bladder, causing a constant disposition to evacuate urine, the *Althœa Officinalis* is a certain remedy; it acts like a charm. It is an important remedy for inflammation of the bladder. A good mode of using it is in form of a warm infusion in doses of a table spoonful every half hour or hour, according to the urgency of the symptoms. The *Althœa Rosa* (Hollyhock) may be used as a substitute, though it is not as good. Every family should cultivate the *Althœa Officinalis* (Marsh Mallow), so that the fresh green root, which is the best, can be procured at any time. I have been able to relieve patients with it, especially females, when all other remedies seemed unavailing. It is particularly useful for urinary difficulties of pregnant females.

Neuralgia.

Aconite and *Bell.* are two important remedies in this affection. If given low, and applied directly along the course of the affected nerves, at full strength of the tincture, [Pg 119] they will almost always effect a cure. The proper way to use them is to give them internally at the second dilution, at intervals of fifteen to thirty minutes, when the pain is severe and nearly constant, and apply *Aconite tincture* as hot as practicable over the course of the nerve, by means of wet cloths, for an hour or two hours, and if the pain has not subsided use *Bell.* locally in the same manner.

If the Neuralgia is periodical, coming on at regular intervals, *Arsenicum* and *China* are the remedies, and they should be used externally as directed for the others, both at the first dilution, and given internally at intervals, in proportion to the violence of the symptoms, the *Arsen.* at the 3d and the *China* at the first dilution. If the patient has used alcoholic drinks to excess, *Nux* is to be used in place of Arsenicum.

Periodical Neuralgia generally requires the same treatment as ague. In females when there is uterine disease, *Pulsatilla* and *Macrotin* are the remedies to be used, as directed above. [Pg 120]

Jaundice.

This disease depends upon derangement of the liver. The skin and whites of the eyes become yellow; the patient grows weak, loses his appetite, is dull and sluggish in all his actions, melancholly and discouraged in his moods.

TREATMENT.

Mercurius and *Podophyllin* given in alternation, each twice a day, will nearly always effect a cure. If the patient is costive, *Nux* should be taken at night, until his bowels become regular.

Bathing the surface daily, or oftener, is a very important measure in the treatment of this affection. As often as once in two or three days, an alkaline bath should be taken. If the patient has fever every day, or once in two days, ever so slight, *China* should be used with *Podophyllin*. If he has been drugged with Mercury in any form, in large doses, even six months or a year before, give *Hydrastin* in place of Mercurius.

Itch.

I shall say but little about this very common and very obstinate affection. Every [Pg 121] body has a "cure for itch" yet nobody cures it short of the use of *Sulphur* in some form. Though the attenuations of Sulphur may sometimes cure itch, it must be acknowledged that such cures are so rare in this country, and the time requisite to accomplish it is so long, as a general rule, that few will trust them.

The most successful remedy, and the one that will always cure quickly, if at all, is *Hepar Sulphurus Potassium*, the common Hepar Sulphur (sulphuret of Potassa) of the shops. To succeed with it most certainly, let the patient be thoroughly bathed with warm soap suds, *quite strong*, in a room at the temperature of 90 to 100°, continuing the bathing and *rubbing* for an hour or more, then dry off the surface with soft cloths, and apply the *Hepar sul.* with water, at the strength of thirty drops of the strong alcoholic solution, with a gill of water, wetting every eruption on the whole surface and let it dry on. This causes some smarting, but it is effectual; it kills the *acarus*, (itch animalcule) and in a few days the sores heal, the itching all subsides immediately. If every pustule has not [Pg 122] been touched, those left may continue to itch, in which case, a second application is necessary. *Hepar Sul.* should be given internally at the third dilution, for a month, once a day, after the baths. Avoid greasy food. For the

Scald Head

of children, where there is a discharge of yellow and watery pus from the sores, and the eruption extends to the ears or face, like the disease called the *crusta lactea* (milk crust), the same washes as for itch, are the most effectual, while at the same time, and for a month or two, the child should have *Hepar Sul.* 5th at night, and *Petroleum* 3d in the morning. Daily ablutions of the head with warm soap suds, and keeping it covered, are absolutely essential.

Carbuncle.

This affection, though it somewhat resembles a common boil, and is by some writers considered only such, in an overgrown state, is, nevertheless, far from being identical with it.

While a *boil* is only a sanitive effort of nature to eliminate the cause of a morbid [Pg 123] process, and tends to a spontaneous, healthy termination, the *carbuncle*, on the contrary, is the very essence of disease; its constant tendency being towards the dissemination of diseased action, causing destruction of the parts affected. It, in fact, appears like a parasite, living by the destruction of surrounding tissues, literally absorbing them and "thriving on death." It begins with a red, livid color, slight aching and burning pains, the part swells and is elevated some like a boil, except that it does not "point," but has a broad base rising like a cone and flattened at the top. It feels soft and spongy, and will appear to fluctuate, but if punctured, blood only flows. The pain and burning increases rapidly, and sooner or later several openings appear upon the top, varying from three or four to half a dozen or more, looking like the holes in a sponge, out of which issues a fluid like thin gruel. Instead of becoming easier after the suppuration begins, as is the case with a boil, the burning increases to an alarming and unbearable extent; cold chills, loss of appetite, great depression of spirits, general nervous [Pg 124] and muscular debility come on. The tumor continues to discharge, turns purple; gangrene beginning in the carbuncle extends to other parts and death follows.

The disease is nearly always confined to quite feeble persons and those past the meridian of life; but I have seen it on younger though feeble patients. It is generally located on the back, occasionally on the head, where it is very dangerous from its liability to affect the brain.

TREATMENT.

If treated very early, *strong tincture of Arnica* applied to the surface of the carbuncle, by cloths wet and laid over the tumor, will often arrest it so that the swelling will not be developed to the suppurative stage. However, to reap any benefit from *Arnica*, it must be applied while the pain is not severe, and the parts only feel bruised and tender to pressure, like a common bruise.

After the ulceration occurs, *Arsenicum* is the great remedy to be relied on. It should be given at the second or third attenuation as often as every three hours, when the pain is severe, and applied to the surface of the [Pg 125] carbuncle freely by cloths laid over it, wet in the first dilution, or by sprinkling the first trituration of the oxyde (1-10) freely upon the open surfaces, so that it may penetrate into the open mouths or orifices. Over this powder apply an emolient poultice, or soft cloths wet in water hot as can be endured. This will soon allay or greatly lessen the pain. It should be repeated as often as any of the burning pain peculiar to the carbuncle returns, until the tumor suppurates in a tolerably healthy manner; then lessen the strength of the *Ars.* applications, and continue them until it has the appearance of a healthy abscess, when only simple dressings are necessary. Some may suppose such strong applications injurious, but I can assure them from abundant experience, that there is not the slightest danger. The carbuncle should *never be punctured* or *cut into*. Such operations always make them worse, and induce a more rapid approach to gangrene.

The patient should have nourishing food, and good native wine may be taken in mod [Pg 126] erate quantities, by a very feeble person, with decided advantage.

Though the knife operations for the removal of carbuncle are always injurious, the chemical effect of *Potash* is frequently most beneficial. I have, in repeated instances, applied to the ulcerated surface, *caustic potash* freely, allowing the dissolved caustic to penetrate to the very "core" by running into the orifices. At first it would produce some smarting, but the pain is different from that of the carbuncle, and the change is agreeable rather than otherwise. Soon after the application all pain ceases, and the tumor, under the use of a poultice, begins to slough off in a few days, leaving a raw surface, disposed to heal kindly. Occasionally, however, the healing process is tardy, when *Arsenicum*, at the third, applied and taken internally, will soon effect a cure.

I have occasionally used *Hepar Sul.* with good effect in the latter stage.

Felon—Whitlow.

For this disease, in the early stage, when the sensation is that of sharp, sticking pain, feeling as though a brier or thistle was in the [Pg 127] finger, immerse the part in water as hot as possible, into which put common salt as long as it will dissolve; hold it in this *hot* salt bath for an hour or more at a time, and when removed, apply finely pulverized salt, wet in *Spirits of Turpentine*; bind on the salt with several thicknesses, and keep it constantly wet with the sp'ts turpt. for twenty-four hours, when, if all symptoms of felon are gone, no further treatment is necessary. As a general rule, the hot bath should be repeated three times a day, especially if the symptoms have existed for several days and there is much pain or swelling, and the dressings should be kept on as above directed for several days, more or less, until all symptoms disappear.

I am quite confident that a large majority, if not all, of the cases if thus treated at any time before pus is formed, will be discussed and cured. If pus has begun to form before the treatment is commenced, this will not *cure* the felon, but it is good treatment, especially the hot bath, as it will greatly lessen the pain. [Pg 128]

By holding it in hot water for an hour or two each day, the suppurative process will be hastened, and as soon as the pus can be felt at any point, fluctuating, puncture and let it out; then continue the hot bath, with *Calendula* (*Marygold*) flowers in the water, keeping the part all the time warm and moist.

For the restless and nervous irritability that frequently occurs, especially in females, *Aconite is the best remedy*. It should be given, one drop of the tincture to a gill of water, in teaspoonful doses, once in one or two hours, and the same applied to the sore. [Pg 129]

DISEASES OF FEMALES

Suppression of the Menses, (Amenorrhœa.)

For sudden suppression from taking cold, as by wetting the feet, there being headache, more or less fever, the pulse frequent and variable, pains in the small of the back and cramp like pains in the pelvic region, give, in alternation, *Aconite* and *Pulsatilla*, as often as every fifteen or twenty minutes in a violent case, and at longer intervals as the patient begins to get easy. Putting the feet into hot water, or taking a hot Sitz bath is very useful. If the patient is sick at the stomach, as is often the case, give lukewarm water freely and let her vomit; after which let her drink freely of water as hot as it can be safely swallowed, adding milk and sugar to make it palatable. The good effects that are often attributed to and experienced from the use of various hot teas in this affection, are, in my opinion, attributable more to the hot fluid alone than to any specific medicinal virtue in the substance of which tea is made. [Pg 130] At all events, very *hot* drink with nothing but water, milk and sugar, is equally efficacious, and my medicine (a few grains of sugar of milk) put into the hot water, seasoned as above, has often obtained great credit, when the *hot water* was alone worthy. Rubbing the loins and abdomen briskly downwards with the hands of a healthy and vigorous nurse, will often excite the menstrual flow after a sudden suppression. If the head is hot, the face full and red, and the arteries of the neck and temples beat violently, give *Bell.* with *Pulsatilla*, and if the lungs are oppressed, use also *Bryonia*, giving the three in rotation. If, after the menstrual flow begins, there is still much pain in the pelvic region, give *Caulophyllin*, which will immediately afford relief.

Apis mel. is very servicable in suppressed menses of several days, or even weeks duration, where there is fever, redness of the face, and pain in the head, and pains in the hips extending to the limbs, especially if there is any tendency to bloating of the abdomen and swelling of the limbs or feet. It acts *promptly* and *efficiently*.

If the suppression has been caused by sudden fright or any strong mental emotion, *Veratrum* should be given in connection with the two former medicines. Should there be great fullness of the vessels of the head, or bleeding at the nose, *Bryonia* with *Pulsatilla* [Pg 131] are to be used. *Bell.* is also useful in this case if the pain in the head is throbbing, especially if any delirium is present.

For suppression in young females, of several months duration, I have used, with much success, *Podophyllin* and *Macrotin*, one at night, the other in the morning, giving them for two or three weeks before the proper time for a return, and a day or two prior to the time, give also *Pulsatilla*, and give the three in rotation, a dose every six hours.

This practice has been successful with me in cases of long standing and apparently obstinate character. Where there is other disease, as an affection of the liver, lungs or stomach, this must be treated and cured, or the menses will not probably return. Great care should be exercised to keep the patient's feet and limbs warm, as upon this may depend her future health.

Dysmenorrhœa.—Painful Menstruation.

For this disorder, I know of no one remedy so valuable as the *Caulophyllin*, but *Pulsatilla* in many cases is efficacious, and as they do not prevent each other's action, I prescribe them in alternation, giving a dose every half hour, for a short time during the paroxysm, or until the pain abates to some extent, then every hour. [Pg 132]

If there is pain in the head, sickness at the stomach, a kind of sick headache, as is often the case, with painful menstruation, *Macrotin* should be used with the others; *Ipecac* is the *Specific* for an excessive flow of the menses with great pain, especially if the stomach is nauseated. It should be given as low as the first dilution, and the tincture, in water, in the proportion of thirty drops to half a pint, injected into the vagina quite warm.

The application of extract of *Belladonna* to the neck of the uterus will often produce immediate and perfect relief. After the patient is relieved from the painful paroxysm, she should be treated so as to prevent a return of the pains at the next monthly period. *Pulsatilla*, *Caulophyllin* and *Podophyllin* are the three medicines that are most certain to effect this object. They are to be given, one medicine each day, a dose at night for three weeks, then morning, noon and night, until the time for the return of the menses, when they should be used oftener if there is pain. If the patient is inclined to be costive, *Nux* should be given at night for a few days before the menstrual period, in place of *Pulsatilla*.

Menorrhagia—Profuse Menses—Flowing.

For this affection, *Ipecac* and *Hamamelis* are the specifics. They should be taken [Pg 133] alternately, at intervals of from half an hour to two hours apart, according to the urgency of the symptoms, and the *Hamamelis* injected into the vagina. These will nearly always arrest the flooding immediately. *Secale* should be used either alone or with the above medicines, if there are bearing down pains like labor pains, and sickness at the stomach in spite of the Ipecac. *Ipecac* alone is often sufficient.

Nursing Sore Mouth.

Sore mouth of nursing women, as the name of the disease indicates, is peculiar to women who are suckling children. It is an inflammation of the mouth, tongue and fauces, which sometimes comes on during pregnancy, several months or but a few days before the birth of the child. It generally, however, makes its first appearance when the child is a few weeks old, and sometimes not till after the lapse of several months. In some cases the tongue and inside of the mouth ulcerate, and the irritation extends to the stomach and bowels, producing distressing and dangerous inflammation of these parts, with severe and obstinate diarrhœa.

For the sore mouth, before diarrhœa begins, give *Eupatorium Aro.* and *Hydrastin*, in alternation, a dose once in three hours, [Pg 134] and wash the mouth with the same, each time. After the diarrhœa occurs, use *Podophyllin* with the other medicines, giving them in rotation, three hours apart. It is best to give a dose of *Podophyllin* night and morning.

I have treated very bad cases of this disease that had been running for more than a year, and been treated with the ordinary remedies directed in the Homœopathic authorities without any permanent benefit, curing them perfectly in ten days with *Podophyllin* and *Leptandrin*, giving them in alternation at the 1st attenuation in half grain doses, at intervals of from four to eight hours according to the frequency of the evacuations. These two remedies are almost certain to arrest *Chronic Dysentery* where there is ulceration of the lower portion of the rectum, a peculiar distress felt at the stomach just before stool, with *sudden* rush of the evacuations and inability to control the inclination even for a few minutes, with a feeling of faintness after the stool.

Leptandrin is the specific for the Dysentery that often succeeds cholera, and these two, *Pod.* and *Lept.*, are almost certain to relieve the "Mexican Diarrhœa," as well as that connected with the fevers along the Mississippi river. [Pg 135]

Mammary Abscess,

(*Ague in the breast – Inflamed breast*.)

This is a disease peculiar to nursing women. The first symptom is a slight pain or soreness in some part of the "breast," which continues to increase for a day or two, when a chill, more or less severe, sets in, followed by high fever and quick pulse, headache and great restlessness. The gland swells and becomes very painful. This is generally a disease of rather slow progress, running eight or ten days and sometimes two or three weeks before abscess forms and "points" to the surface.

TREATMENT.

Phosphorus is to be taken internally, and the first dilution put in water, twenty drops to one gill, and applied to the surface by means of cloths wet in the mixture, as hot as it can be borne, and laid over the whole breast. If this is done and the medicine given internally every hour, as early as the first and frequently as late as the second or third day, it is quite sure to remove the disease and prevent an abscess. It is best to use it even much later. In fact it often succeeds as late as the fifth or sixth day, and if it does not prevent the abscess, it so far palliates the severe symptoms as to render the pain but slight and keep the patient comfortable. [Pg 136]

An application of the Tincture of Cantharides diluted with water and applied to the breast by cloths wet in it, to the extent of producing considerable redness and even eruptions, and the second dilution of the same taken in drop doses every three hours, has proved successful in subduing the inflammation after *Phos.* had failed, and it was supposed an abscess would form in spite of any treatment.

I recently succeeded in giving perfect relief with *Apis Mel.* internally, applying it externally after the pain and swelling was very great. I am of opinion that the *Apis* is a valuable remedy.

After abscess forms as soon as the pus can be felt at any point, soft and fluctuating under the skin, *puncture* and let it out, then poultice it for a few days until it heals, giving *Phosphorus* and applying it to the sore. In *puncturing*, always be *very particular* to have the lancet or knife enter so that the edge will look towards the point of the nipple, so as not to cut *across* the milk ducts, which all run toward that point, and if cut off will close up so that the milk which may be secreted at any future time cannot get out, and swelling, pain and severe inflammation, abscess and ulceration will be the consequence; whereas, if the cut is made lengthwise of the ducts, very few, if any will be cut off, and all future danger [Pg 137] will be avoided. Apply an elm poultice from the beginning to the end of treatment. For malignant ulcers of the breasts, the *Cornus Sericea* is a most potent remedy. It is to be taken internally at the first dilution, and applied in strong infusion or diluted *Tr.* of the bark to the sore.

Sore Nipples.

This affection of nursing women frequently comes on before the birth of the child, but generally does not make its appearance until after the suckling has continued for a week or more. It seems in some cases to be connected with the aphthæ (sore mouth) of the child, or at least to be aggravated by contact with the sore mouth; on the other hand it sometimes seems as though the sore nipples produced the sore mouth of the child.

TREATMENT.

I treat both the nipple and the child's mouth with the same remedy *Eupatorium aro.*, applied at the strength of 6 drops of the tincture, to a teaspoonful of water, the application being made by a soft cloth, wet and laid over the nipple; give drop doses of the same strength internally every three hours, which will, in nearly all cases effect a cure in one or two days. The child's mouth should be wet with the same [Pg 138] each time just before nursing. The oil from the pit of the butter nut, (Juglan's Cinerea,) obtained by heating the pit and pressing out the oil, applied to the nipple, will generally cure it after 3 or 4 applications about six hours apart. The child may take hold when the oil is on, without danger. This remedy is sufficient in nearly all cases.

Leucorrhœa and Prolapsus Uteri—Whites, Female Weakness.

The disease depends in all cases upon *inflammation* of the uterus, or vagina, or both.

The inflammation may be simply in the neck of the uterus extending to the posterior surface of the vagina, or the latter may not be affected; or it may extend to the whole internal surface of the uterus, producing swelling of that organ, both the fundus and neck.

The swelling may be confined mostly to the fundus, causing it to be too large for the space it ordinarily fills, hence there will be more or less *displacement* of the womb, and crowding upon other parts, as the bladder or rectum. In some cases, the swelling is more on one side than on the other, so that it will be crowded over to the opposite side. These displacements are often called *prolapsus uteri*, or "*falling of the womb*," [Pg 139] carrying the idea that the difficulty depends upon a morbid relaxation of the ligaments that support the organ. Not one case in a hundred is of this latter character, but nearly, if not all, depend upon the inflammation and swelling above mentioned. How futile then, not to say *hurtful*, must be all instruments for, and all attempts at replacing and supporting it by *force*! All such mechanical meddling is injurious, and should, with all the "supporters," be condemned and discarded.

They may afford temporary relief, but this is at the expense of future health. Cure the disease, relieve the inflammation, and nature will replace the organ. Leucorrhœa is always present where there is ulceration of the neck of the womb, and this ulcerated condition exists to a greater or less extent, in many cases where it is not suspected by the patient. It is vastly more prevalent than is generally supposed. The *symptoms* are numerous. Among the more prominent are a sense of weight and bearing down in the pelvis, pains extending down the limbs, aching and weakness of the small of the back, headache, more or less gastric disturbance, dyspepsia, the food souring on the stomach. There is often, especially when there are ulcers on the parts, a distressing sense of heat or a smarting sensation. The menstrual function is [Pg 140] frequently deranged, the bowels costive, the urethra, by being pressed, becomes irritable and burns and smarts whenever the urine is evacuated. The sleep is disturbed and unrefreshing, and the whole nervous system is unstrung.

The discharge from the diseased surfaces, in an ordinary case without ulceration, is of a mucous or muco-purulent character, not unlike an ordinary catarrhal secretion. When ulceration exists it is dark, fetid or bloody, or sanious and purulent, sometimes it is acrid, excoriating the parts.

TREATMENT.

Inflammation or ulceration, either acute or chronic, in these parts does not differ essentially in its characteristics from the same affection in other mucous surfaces.

The proper treatment for a catarrh of other mucous surfaces will be applicable to these, though there is no doubt but that some medicines are more specifically adapted to these than to other organs.

In the early stage of the complaint, while the inflammation is acute, or sub-acute, the discharge thin or white, *Copaiva* and *Macrotin* are to be given once in 6 hours alternately. During the same time let injections into the vagina of warm soap and water be used twice a day, to cleanse the parts of the secretion, followed in half an [Pg 141] hour by a wash of warm water, into which *tr. of Macrotys* has been put in proportion of 40 drops to half a pint. The application should be made with an 8 ounce or at least 6 ounce curved pipe syringe, so as to throw it with considerable force. If there is a burning sensation, use the washes quite warm, until the heat of the parts is allayed. Avoid the use of *cold* injections as long as any inflammation exists. If the bearing down is present with burning in the parts, *Bell.* is to be used in rotation with the two former remedies. If the sensation is that of smarting, *Cantharis* is to be used in place of Bell.

Where the disease comes on soon after child-birth, *Podophyllin is the Specific*. It is to be given at the first attenuation three times daily in half gr. doses of the trituration. In this case let the parts be freely washed daily with a solution of borax, quite warm. In the *chronic* form of the disease, especially where *barrenness* exists, *Macrotin*,

Podophyllin and *Hydrastin*, given morning, noon and night, in the order named, will, in nearly all cases, afford relief.

For females who have never borne children, give *Phos. acid*, 2d and *Eryrgium Aquaticum* 1, night and morning for a week, and then give them at the 3d dilution until the symptoms subside. If there are headache and derangement of [Pg 142] the stomach, *Macrotin* and *Podophyllin* should be used, each once a day, between the latter remedies. When the discharge is colored and the pains darting, cutting or smarting, indicating ulceration, or if ulceration is discovered by examination, use *Macrotin* and *Hydrastin* internally, injecting the latter upon the affected parts freely. The ulcerated surfaces should be well washed off every day with soap and water, or a solution of borax, and the medicine (*Hydrastin*) in form of infusion, used half an hour after the other wash. If the neck of the womb looks dark, and is ulcerated, or is hard and painful to the touch, especially on probing the cavity, *Cornus Sericea* must be used both as a wash to the parts, and at the first dilution internally, using them twice a day. This remedy will often cure malignant cases.

It takes a long time in some instances to cure a chronic case, but if persevered in, these remedies will not be likely to fail. [2]

[Pg 143]

Morning Sickness of Pregnant Females.

The most efficient and certain remedy for this symptom is *Macrotin*. It should be taken at the first attenuation, a dose before rising in the morning, and one every six hours during the day, as long as the sickness is troublesome. It will generally relieve in a few days. If the stomach is sour use *Pulsatilla* with the *Macrotin*.

As a *preparation for labor*, a dose (one grain) of *Macrotin* at the first attenuation given in the morning, and the same of *Caulophyllin* at evening, is of great service.

Whatever others may think or say in relation to any preparatory treatment for labor, I have reason to know as well as anything in medicine be known, that patients treated as here directed, pass through labor much quicker, frequently in one-fourth the usual time. Their sufferings are comparatively trifling, and the length of time for recovery to ordinary health after labor is abridged from three-fourths to nine-tenths that of former labors. I am quite confident that the medicines produced this difference.

For *irregularity of labor pains*, and for distressing *after pains*, the *Caulophyllin* is specific.

During labor it should be given at the 2d attenuation in about half grain doses, every half hour, until the pains are regular. Two or three doses at most, and generally one will suffice.

For the after pains it may be given in alternation with *Ipecac* or *Aconite* if there is flooding, or with *Pulsatilla* when the flooding is not troublesome, a dose once in half an hour, until the pains are checked.

For *Rigidity* of the soft parts and severe, *retarded and long protracted labor*, where the pains are strong and irregular, and great pain and exhaustion is experienced on account of the unyielding condition of the parts, *Lobelia Inflata* given in drop doses of the tr. in water, once in twenty minutes, in alternation with *Caulophyllin* as above directed, will in a short time produce the proper condition of the parts, while they render the pains stronger, regular and progressive.

In urgent cases I have given the medicines every 5 or 10 minutes, with decided benefit.

A Useful Hint to Mothers.

Children push beans, peas, corn, &c., into the nose and ear, causing much alarm. To remove such a body take a syringe that works tightly, put the end of the pipe against the bean, shot, or other substance, draw back the piston so as to *suck* up the article firmly as the pipe is withdrawn from the cavity. [Pg 145]

LOCAL APPLICATIONS.

That medicines act locally, that is, manifest their symptoms by peculiar derangement or disturbance of some particular part of the system, more prominently than of any other part, for the time, no one will deny. That each one has some particular locality or tissue upon which its action is more perceptible than anywhere else, is equally undeniable, and that the prominent symptoms are often external and local, is also true. Yet, with these truths clearly demonstrated, there are those of our school who discard the external or local application of all remedies except *Arnica*.

Why this is done, is difficult to determine, unless we can believe that such physicians suppose it to be *heresy* to make use of any remedy in a different manner from what was recommended by the "Father of Homœopathy," and abjure all possibility of *improvement* in our practice.

That nearly if not all medicines, may be applied externally with advantage, when there are local manifestations similar to those produced by the drugs, there can be no doubt in the mind of any sensible man. That they will act favorably when so used is *reasonable*, as a matter of theory, and that they do, as a matter of fact, has been *proven* to my mind, by abundant experience in their use. Therefore, I hesitate not to recommend the practice [Pg 146] to others. Medicines must act either by combination with the affected part, or by *Catalysis*, changing the molecular action of the living tissues. In either case, they must come directly in contact with the part to be affected. This *must* be done through the circulation, when taken internally, or it *may* be done by direct application of the remedy to the diseased tissue, when that is so situated as to be reached. The difference is greatly in favor of the latter mode when that is practicable, from the greater certainty of its results. This assertion is based, not upon vague hypothesis, but upon *actual practice*.

Entertaining these views, however heretical they may be pronounced, I shall proceed to mention some of the remedies I have learned to use thus, and the cases for which they are prescribed. I would remark that, in selecting a remedy, it must be done with as much certainty of its homœopathic relation to the local or general symptoms for external as for internal use. I have found, however, that much lower attenuations are requisite and admissible.

Arnica is highly applicable to *bruises*, and is valuable also when applied to lacerated or mangled surfaces, to the surface of the limb where a bone is fractured, also about the joint when it has been dislocated. It is to be used in the form of *Arnicated water*, by putting one or two drops to a gill of water [Pg 147] for application where the skin is ruptured or the surface raw, and ten to twenty drops to the gill, upon parts where the skin is sound. It is useful also, for *boils*, and *carbuncles* in the *early stage*, the *strong tincture* to be applied when the surface is sound, and (to boils) when the surface is open, one drop to a gill of water.

Aconite

Is applicable to inflamed eyes, in the early stage, where the disease is in the conjunctiva, (that portion which lines the lids and covers the front of the ball), especially if there is a sense of scratching, as though some foreign substance is in the eye, great intolerance of light, chilly sensations, with more or less fever, and quick pulse. Put three or four drops to a gill of warm water, and apply it freely.

It is also very valuable for *Neuralgia*, applied strong and warm, along the course, or at the origin of the affected nerve. In neuralgia of the face, apply it upon the side of the face, also just behind and below the ear of the affected side.

It is of much value as a remedy for neuralgic affections of the womb. I have relieved the most distressing symptoms of neuralgia of the womb, in a few minutes, by injecting warm water containing twenty to forty drops of *tr. Aconite* to the pint. By repeating this application at every paroxysm, [Pg 148] patients recover rapidly, each succeeding attack being lighter, and the interval between being longer, until they cease entirely. It may be used with much benefit in the same manner, for *Hysteritis*, as well as recent cases of *Leucorrhœa*. It is the most valuable remedy applied to the *Eye* for a *wound* of that organ.

In *Gonorrhœa*, it is more valuable as a local remedy, than most of those now in use. It will frequently cure alone. In this case, it is to be used with an equal part of the *tr.* and warm water.

Belladonna

has great power as a local remedy in *Erysipelas*, to be applied with water in proportion of ten drops of the *tr.* to a gill of warm water. It is also of much value applied to the surface of inflamed breasts; also injected when there is inflammation of the *uterus*, with pressing pains as though the bowels would be pressed out. *Very valuable* in parturition where there is rigidity of the *os uteri*, with fullness of the head and throbbing of the temples. It has the specific power to relax circular fibres without affecting the longitudinal.

Calendula,

is applied to wounds, *incised* and *lacerated*, promoting healing by the first intention. It is a valuable application for wounds in [Pg 149] scrofulous persons, which tend to suppurate rather than heal by the first intention. It is also useful in old sores.

The *Calendula Cerate* is one of the best of dressings for any abraded surface.

Conium

is valuable as a *palliative* upon cancerous tumors. As a *curative remedy* it is useful in chronic ophthalmia, especially the purulent of children; useful also for *indurated* swellings.

Thuya

is a specific when locally used for *Sycosis*, also for fungoid cancerous tumors. I have cured well-marked cases of *Fungus Hæmatodes* with the tinct. Thuya applied to the surface of the tumor.

The *Thuja Cerate* is a valuable application for malignant ulcers.

Cornus Sericea

will often cure malignant ulcers both of the breast and uterus, used as a wash.

Arsenicum

acts favorably on cancers, and is a specific when applied to the surface of *carbuncle*.

Ipecac

acts very beneficially when applied to the surface where there is high fever, with nausea and vomiting. Half an ounce of *tr.* Ipecac to two quarts of tepid water, applied with a sponge to the whole surface, acts like [Pg 150] magic in yellow fever, allaying the nausea, producing free and health-restoring perspiration.

Rhus Tox,

applied, with water at the strength of thirty drops of the *tr.* to a gill, to parts affected with *Rheumatism*, acts very beneficially. It is also a most valuable application at half the above strength upon parts affected with Erysipelas, when the surface is swollen, and there are vessicles filled with fluid like a blister in burns.

It is also useful for sores that exist as the chronic effects of burns when the proper treatment had not been used in the beginning, and the healing process was never perfected.

Rhus Cerate is a very useful application to irritable ulcers.

Hepar Sulphur

is a specific for *Itch and Scald Head,* applied in form of a wash with twenty to thirty drops of *tr. Hepar Sul.* to a gill of water. Also for ill-conditioned scrofulous ulcers, generally.

Cuprum Aceticum.

(*Acetate of Copper Verdigris*) applied to *Cancerous* ulcers of the face, *Lupus* or *Noli-me-tangere*, in the early stage, will in most cases effect a perfect cure, especially if for a week previously the part has been [Pg 151] wet daily with *tr. Thuja*. The best mode of applying the *acetate* is to mix the impalpable powder, as prepared for paint, with some substance to form a cerate, as equal parts of bees-wax and mutton suet, with 1-50 to 1-100 part of the pure *acetate* as found in the bottom of the can, when prepared in oil for paint; heat all together and stir until cool. This forms a good plaster for covering and shielding the sore while its medicinal property is in the *Cuprum Aceticum* diluted as above. It is quite useful for any ill conditioned ulcer.

Acetic Acid

is a most efficient remedy applied to old irritable *varicose ulcers* on the limbs of females who have suffered from *Phlegmasia Dolens*, (milk leg.)

It may be applied as a wash to the part once or twice a day at the strength of 1-20th of the acid with water, or in the form of good cider vinegar.

The manufactured vinegar of the cities does *not* usually contain acetic acid.

Arum Triphyllum is a specific to allay the inflammation and excessive pain in *scrofulous swellings* of the neck, (*Kings Evil*.) The pure drug in powder, wet with warm water, or the green root bruised so as to form a poultice, is to be applied over the swelling. It soon discusses the swelling, [Pg 152] or if pus has already formed, allays the the pain, and brings the pus to the surface, and if continued, disposes it to heal rapidly.

Baptisia Tinctoria applied as a poultice either in the powdered drug, or with some other substance wet with the infusion or *tr.*, *arrests gangrene* in a short time. It is especially useful for threatened or actual gangrene arising from *lacerated* wounds or scalds with wounds, as in accidents connected with the explosion of steam boilers; when we often have scalds and lacerations in the same wound.

Hydrastus Canadensis used as a gargler in a putrid state of the throat in malignant *Scarlet fever*, arrests the destructive process *at once*.

It is also a most excellent application for inflamed eyes in the second or sub-acute stage.

PROPHYLACTICS.

(*Preventives of Disease.*)

TO PREVENT SCARLET FEVER

Give Belladonna at the 3d attenuation, three to six pellets, according to the age of the child, every morning, during the prevalence of the epidemic. This is for the common or mild form of the disease. If the prevailing epidemic is of the *malignant* kind, producing fatal ulcerations of the throat, give *Bell.* once [Pg 153] in two days and *Mercurius Corrosivus* at the 3d attenuation on the alternate day.

While *Bell.* is a very certain preventive of the common eruptive Scarlatina, it is not as certain to prevent the *malignant* form. Though it renders the latter much more mild, the *Merc. Cor.* is necessary to ward it off entirely, or so modify as to divest it of the dangerous features.

TO PREVENT YELLOW FEVER

Take *Aconite*, *Belladonna* and *Macrotin*, 1st in rotation one dose a day. If there is any headache, or pains occur in other parts of the body, or a languid feeling, take a dose twice or three times a day in rotation.

TO PREVENT BILIOUS FEVER OR AGUE

Take *Podophyllin*, *Baptisia* and *Gelseminum* 1st in rotation, one dose at night, and if symptoms of fever, as headache and loss of appetite, or bad taste in the mouth in the morning appear, take a dose three times a day, and refrain entirely from food for one or two days.

TO PREVENT TYPHOID FEVER

When exposed, as in nursing the sick, take *Baptisia* 2d, and *Macrotin* 2d, a dose three times a day.

TO PREVENT SMALL-POX

Use *Macrotin* 1st night and morning, and if nursing or exposed frequently, use it every four hours.

TO PREVENT CHOLERA.

Camphor (*pellets medicated* with the pure tincture) *Veratrum* 3d, and *Arsenicum* 3d, [Pg 154] should be taken in rotation—a dose morning, noon and night, in the order named; so as to take a dose of each every twenty-four hours. If any sense of weakness or trembling comes on, use the *Camphor* oftener; if pain or uneasiness in the bowels threatening diarrhœa, use the *Veratrum*, and for increased thirst with uneasiness at the stomach *Arsenicum* more frequently.

TO PREVENT DIARRHŒA

Where it is prevailing as an *epidemic*, *Ipecac* at night, and *Veratrum* in the morning will often *suffice*. For *teething children* give *Ipecac* and *Chamomilla* in the same manner.

TO PREVENT DYSENTERY

In hot weather when bilious diseases prevail, use *Mercurius* 3d, *Podophyllin* 2d, and *Leptandrin* 1st in rotation, giving one dose a day.

In the winter, or when *Typhoid fevers* prevail, use *Mercurius* and *Rhus* tox. alternately a dose every day.

TO PREVENT ITCH.

A dose of *Sulphur*, or rubbing a little flour of sulphur on the hands, will generally suffice.

TO PREVENT COLDS

Keep the *arms*, *hands* and *chest* well clothed and warm. *Affecting* the *head* as *catarrh*, or the pelvic regions keep the *feet and ancles warm and dry*. Affecting joints and muscles as Rheumatism—protect the *Spine* (back) from colds and currents of air. [Pg 155]

After an accidental exposure as by getting the feet wet, or being caught in a shower, drink *bountifully* of cold water, and take a dose of *Nux*; followed in an hour by *Aconite*, if any chilliness is felt, or *Copaiva* if the head is "stuffed up."

In winter and spring when the weather is mild, but there is snow, or the ground is damp, more clothes are necessary than when it is freezing hard and the air is dry.

PREPARATION OF MEDICINE.

As it often becomes necessary for the practitioner to make more or less of his own dilutions and attenuations, some brief instructions especially to new beginners, may not come amiss.

Medicine is prepared by mixing it with distilled water, or purified 98 per cent. Alcohol; or if solid and dry, by reducing it to powder and triturating (rubbing) it in a mortar with pure sugar or Sugar of Milk. The liquid is called *dilution*, the powder *trituration*. The attenuations are mostly made at the decimal (1-10,) or centecimal (1-100) ratio and numbered 1, 2, 3, &c., by putting ten drops of the liquid with ninety drops of Alcohol, or ten grains of the powder with ninety grains of Sugar for the 1st, and ten grains or drops of the 1st with ninety more of Alcohol or Sugar, as the case may be, for the 2nd, and so on to any desirable extent. [Pg 156]

If the centecimal attenuation is adopted, one grain or drop is used instead of ten, as in the decimal.

I prefer the decimal to the centecimal ratio. Not that there can possibly be any difference in the action of the medicines, at the same attenuation, whether it was brought to that state through a series of 1-10, or 1-100; the 3d at the 1-100 ratio of dilution being *precisely the same* as the 6th at 1-10. My preference for the decimal ratio is based upon the greater convenience and accuracy of measuring larger quantities.

Accuracy is very desirable, but the practice of *guessing* at the amount as pursued by some, is anything but accurate. When one makes his dilutions by putting the fluid into a vial and "*pouring it all out,*" *guessing* that he has a *drop* left which is to medicate the ninety-nine drops of Alcohol or water, he may put in by guess, I am inclined to *guess* that he knows nothing, *accurately* as to what dilution he is making. (See Hull's Laura, introduction, also Jahr & Possart's Pharmacopœia and Posology.) For if the vial is small and quite smooth there may not be a drop left, or if it is rough, there may be several drops.

Yet some physicians make their dilutions thus, and insist upon the superiority of the centecimal over the decimal attenuations.

Whatever ratio is adopted, should be *accurately* followed. Have true scales for weighing solids, and a graduated measure marked from ten drops up to one hundred for liquids; then [Pg 157] *always* weigh or measure *accurately* the medicine, as well as the substance with which it is to be attenuated.

The measure and mortar, after using them for one medicine, can be cleaned preparatory for another, with scalding water, rinsing them with purified Alcohol, then drying.

Never smoke or chew Tobacco in any place, but if you are such a *slave* to habit, that you must do it despite your good sense and better judgment, never do either, or have tobacco or any other odoriferous substance about your person when you are preparing medicines, or they are exposed to the air. Keep the medicines excluded from the light and air as far as practicable.

Triturate the powders thoroughly for an hour or more upon each, and shake the dilution from fifty to one hundred times, more for the higher attenuations.

It is better to medicate pellets in large bottles, filling them half or two-thirds full, put in just liquid enough to wet every one, but not so as to dissolve any. Shake them until all are equally wet, and let them stand for four or five days, if practicable, shaking them up two or three times a day until all are dry.

APPENDIX

On the Use of Gelseminum Semp. in Fevers. By J. S. Douglas, A. M., M. D., Prof. of Mat. Med. and Special Pathology, in the Western Homœpathic College, Cleveland; author of "Treatment of Intermittents," &c.

Such has been the general result of the treatment of the fevers of this country, that most Homœopathic physicians deny the possibility of *breaking up* a fever when once established.

Those who labor under this impression, will be soon convinced of the error by properly employing the *Gelseminum semper virens*, or yellow Jasmine. Having proved this drug repeatedly on myself and seven or eight others, it was impossible to avoid the conviction that it would be homœopathic to the ordinary fevers of this country.

The pathogenetic symptoms, almost uniformly experienced, are the following, the dose being from one to five drops:

Within a few minutes, sometimes within two or three, a marked depression of pulse, which becomes 10, 15 or 20 beats less in the minute, if quiet, but greatly disturbed by movement. Chilliness, especially along the back, pressive pain of the head, most generally of the temples, sometimes in the occiput, at others, over the head. The chilliness is soon followed by a glow of heat and prickling of the skin, and quickly succeeded by perspiration which is sometimes profuse and disposed to be persistent, continuing from twelve to twenty-four hours. As soon as the re-action takes place after the chill, the pulse rises as much above the normal standard, as it was before depressed below it. With these symptoms is a puffy, swollen look and feeling of the eye-lids, slimy and disagreeable or bitter taste in the mouth, languid feeling of the back and limbs, and sleepiness.

As example affords the best illustration, we will give one to illustrate the usual action of this drug in fevers:

P. W., aged 21, sanguine temperament, had been complaining of languor, and want of appetite for three weeks. For a week has been unable to attend to business. Took a cathartic, and was, of course, worse. For the last thirty-six hours had been seriously sick. June 30, 1858, had the following symptoms: Pulse rather full, but weak and vascillating, about 100 per minute. Tongue red and dry; hands tremulous when extending them; tongue trembles when protruded; the mind wanders; he reaches after imaginary objects; lips dry and parched; he is uneasy, restless. Now this, all will recognize as a case which had been long in coming on, and was fairly established, and was not likely to be *broken up* by ordinary means. He took one drop of *Gelseminum tincture* to be repeated every hour, if needed. The next morning he reported that he had been in a perspiration ever since fifteen minutes after taking the first dose, had slept quietly during the night, the tongue and lips were moist, mind clear, pulse 80, and steady. The next day I found him dressed and down stairs, with good appetite and free from disease. I could give sixty cases of equally prompt results from this precious drug, in fevers which make their attack rather suddenly, whether from cold or otherwise, and attended with chilliness, pain in the limbs, head and back, variously disordered taste of the mouth, with great restlessness. The almost uniform effect, in these cases is, a cessation of the chills, within from two to five minutes, quickly followed by a glow of heat and prickling of the surface; and within from five to twenty minutes, perspiration with progressive abatement of all the pains and restlessness. The patient falls asleep, and after a longer or shorter time, wakes with a consciousness that his disease is *broken up*—and this proves to be the truth. Like all other drugs, the dose must be various, generally one drop repeated every half hour, till the desired effect is produced repeated afterwards as occasion may require.

In simple cases of fever, I regard it as *the* remedy, not only, but *the only* remedy required. There are, of course, many cases of fever, with local complications, as inflammation of the liver, &c., &c., where other remedies will be necessary. Half a drop, or even a quarter, is often sufficient. The largest I have yet given is five drops, and this in only one case.

Several Homœopathic physicians to whom I have recommended it, have made equally favorable reports of it.

My experience has been, that not a few of our Western fevers, especially if neglected beyond the incipient stages, are accompanied by such gastric and bilious disorder, as to require *Mercurius*, *China*, or *Podophyllin*, after the general febrile symptoms are removed by *Gels.* But at an early stage, the *Gels.* alone will prevent the development of these complications.

The drug seems to me to act specifically and energetically, not only upon the circulatory system, but equally so upon the nervous system, allaying nervous irritability more effectually in fevers, than *Coff.*, *Cham.*, *Bell.*, *Nux*, or any other drug we possess. As it acts very quickly, the first dose may be soon repeated and increased, if no effect is observed.

FOOTNOTES

[1] Note.—The Eclectic Physicians use equal parts of Quinine and Prussiate of Iron, with marked success in agues, giving from one to three grains of the mixture at a dose, every two hours, or oftener, for ten or twelve hours, and some times more, during the intermission. An intelligent Homœopathic Physician informs me that he has used with *uniform* success, a *trituration* of this mixture of Quinine and Prussiate of Iron, in proportion of ten grains of the Sugar of Milk to one of the Mixture, giving the trituration in doses of about one grain

every hour through the chill, fever and intermission. Very few cases had a second chill after taking the prescription. I have used this trituration successfully in a few cases.

[2] Note.—The late Prof. Morrow was remarkably successful, and became justly celebrated for curing hard cases of Leucorrhœa ulceration and "Prolapsus uteri."

Almost his entire reliance in their treatment were the *Macrotys* and *Caulophyllum*, given internally and by injection upon the parts. He gave the Macrotys in the form of tincture every day to the extent of producing specific head symptoms when he discontinued it till the next day, using the Caulophyllum in the meantime in small doses. He rarely if ever failed.